Redesigning the Health Care Team
Diabetes Prevention and Lifelong Management

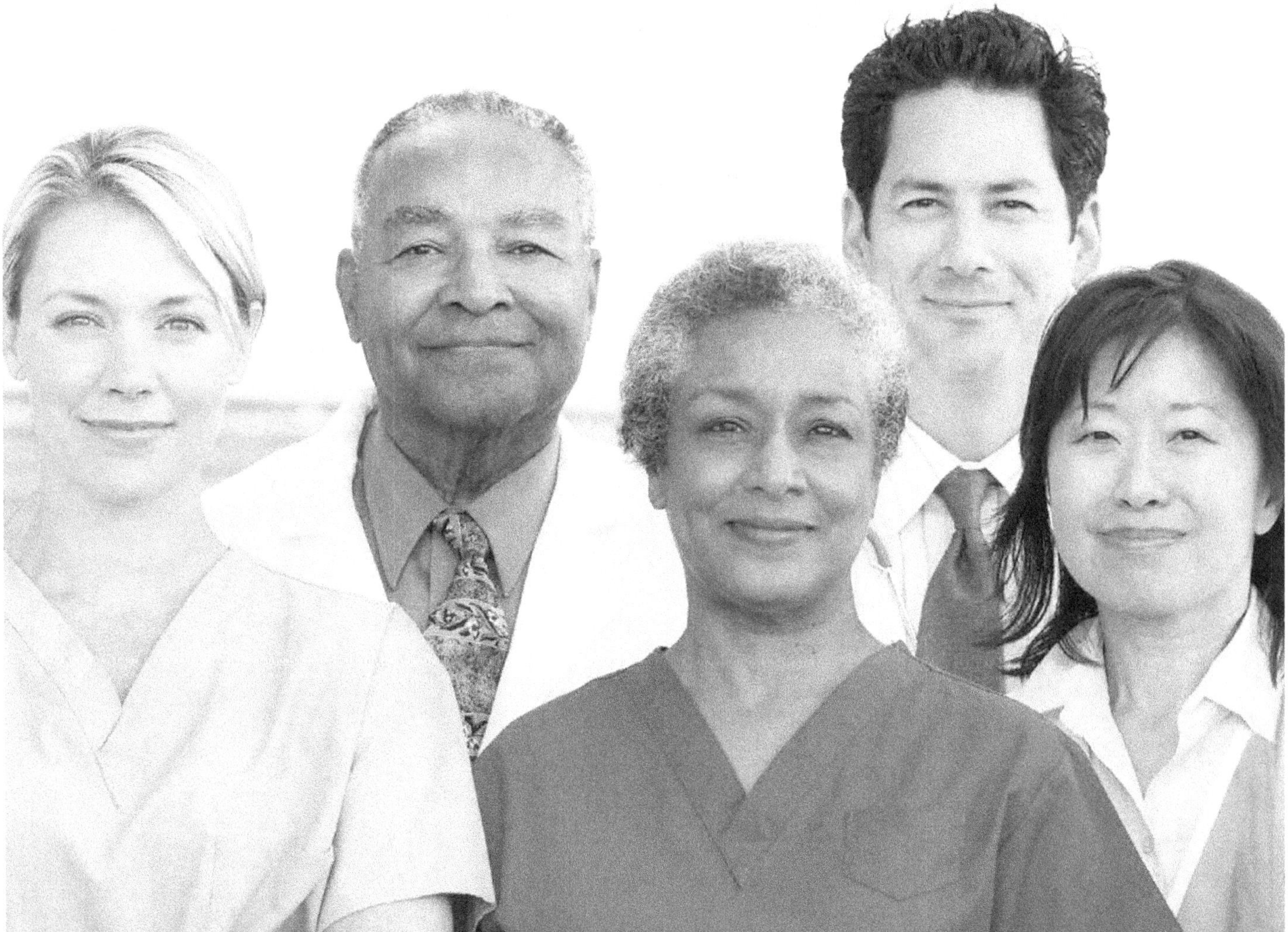

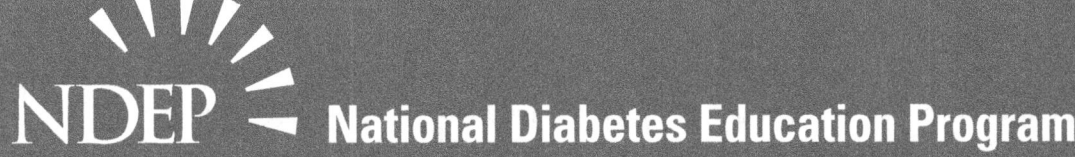

NDEP National Diabetes Education Program

A program of the National Institutes of Health and the Centers for Disease Control and Prevention

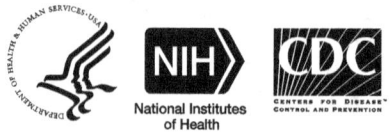

The U.S. Department of Health and Human Services' National Diabetes Education Program (NDEP) is jointly sponsored by the National Institutes of Health and the Centers for Disease Control and Prevention with the support of more than 200 partner organizations.

www.YourDiabetesInfo.org   1-888-693-NDEP (1-888-693-6337)   TTY: 1-866-569-1162

NIH Publication No. 13-7739   NDEP-37   Last Reviewed February 2013

Table of Contents

Credits and Acknowledgments

The U.S. Department of Health and Human Services' National Diabetes Education Program (NDEP) is jointly sponsored by the National Institutes of Health and the Centers for Disease Control and Prevention, with the support of more than 200 partner organizations. The NDEP involves public and private partners in activities designed to improve treatment and outcomes for people with diabetes, promote early diagnosis, and ultimately prevent the onset of this serious and costly disease. These partnerships help to make NDEP goals a reality. The NDEP greatly appreciates the expertise of the following people and hereby acknowledges their contributions to the development of this guide.

CONTENT ADVISORY GROUP

W. Lee Ball, Jr., O.D., F.A.A.O.
American Optometric Association

Mary Jo Goolsby, Ed.D., M.S.N., N.P-C., F.A.A.N.P.
American Academy of Nurse Practitioners

Amy Nicholas, Pharm.D.
American Pharmacists Association

Amparo Gonzalez, R.N., C.D.E., F.A.A.D.E.
American Association of Diabetes Educators

M. Sue Kirkman, M.D.
American Diabetes Association

Patti Urbanski, M.Ed., R.D., L.D., C.D.E.
Academy of Nutrition and Dietetics

WRITER/EDITOR

Elizabeth Warren-Boulton, R.N., M.S.N.
Hager Sharp, Inc., Washington, DC

REVIEWERS

NDEP Executive Committee

Ann Albright, Ph.D., R.D.
Division of Diabetes Translation, Centers for Disease Control and Prevention

Lawrence Blonde, M.D.
Chief of Endocrinology and Metabolic Diseases and Vice Chairman of Medicine at the Ochsner Clinic in New Orleans

Jeff Caballero, M.P.H.
Association of Asian Pacific Community Health Organizations

Judith Fradkin, M.D.
Division of Diabetes, Endocrinology, and Metabolic Diseases, National Institute of Diabetes and Digestive and Kidney Diseases, National Institutes of Health

Martha M. Funnell, M.S., R.N., C.D.E.
Former Chair, National Diabetes Education Program Michigan Diabetes Research and Training Center

NDEP Partner Representatives
Kristina Ernst, R.N., C.D.E., Division of Diabetes Translation, Centers for Disease Control and Prevention

NDEP Health Care Professional Work Group Members
Barbara Bartman, M.D., M.P.H.; John Buse, M.D., Ph.D.; Michael Gonzalez-Campoy, M.D., Ph.D., F.A.C.E.; Joe Humphey, M.D.; Bob McNellis, P.A., M.P.H.; Suzen M. Moeller, M.D., Ph.D.; Michael Parchman, M.D., M.P.H., F.A.A.F.P.; Sandy Parker, R.D., C.D.E.; Leonard Pogach, M.D., M.B.A.; Kathy Tuttle, M.D, F.A.S.N., F.A.C.P.

NDEP Directors

Joanne Gallivan, M.S., R.D.
Director, National Diabetes Education Program, National Institute of Diabetes and Digestive and Kidney Diseases, National Institutes of Health

Diane Tuncer, B.S.
Deputy Director, National Diabetes Education Program, National Institute of Diabetes and Digestive and Kidney Diseases, National Institutes of Health

Jude McDivitt, Ph.D.
Director, National Diabetes Education Program, Division of Diabetes Translation, Centers for Disease Control and Prevention

Betsy Rodriguez, R.N., M.S.N., C.D.E.
Deputy Director, National Diabetes Education Program, Division of Diabetes Translation, Centers for Disease Control and Prevention

NDEP Pharmacy, Podiatry, Optometry, and Dental Professionals Work Group Members
Meg D. Atwood, R.D.H., M.P.S.; Dennis R. Frisch, D.P.M.; Martin Gillis, D.D.S., M.A.Ed.; Philip T. Rodgers, Pharm.D., B.C.P.S., C.D.E., C.P.P., F.C.C.P.; Don Zettervall, R.Ph., C.D.E., C.D.M.

NDEP Diabetes in Children and Adolescents Work Group Members
Nichole Bobo, R.N., M.S.N., A.N.P.; Ryan Brown, M.D., F.A.A.P.; Jane K. Kadohiro, Dr.P.H., A.P.R.N., C.D.E.; Mary Pat King, M.S.; Barbara Linder, M.D.; Katie Marschilok, R.N., C.D.E., BC-ADM; Laura Shea, R.N., C.D.E.; Janet Silverstein, M.D.

Executive Summary

This guide is designed to help health care professionals and health care organizations implement collaborative, multidisciplinary team care for adults and children with diabetes in a variety of settings. Collaborative teams that provide continuous, supportive, and effective care for people with diabetes throughout the course of their disease are a model for the prevention and management of chronic diseases. Well-implemented diabetes team care can be cost-effective and the preferred method of care delivery, particularly when services include health promotion and disease prevention, in addition to intensive clinical management. Team care is a key component of health care reform initiatives that incorporate an integrated health care delivery system, especially those for chronic disease prevention and management.

Diabetes is a serious, common, and costly disease that affects 25.8 million Americans, or 8.3 percent of the U.S. population. About 90 to 95 percent of people with diabetes have type 2, which usually occurs in adults over age 45 but is increasingly occurring in younger age groups. Type 1 is usually diagnosed during childhood, although adults can also develop the disease. Some patients may have features of both type 1 and type 2 diabetes, which further complicates disease treatment and management. In addition, at least 79 million U.S. adults have prediabetes, which places them at increased risk for cardiovascular disease and type 2 diabetes. The chronic complications of diabetes (cardiovascular disease, vision loss, kidney failure, nerve damage, and lower-extremity amputations) result in higher rates of disability, increased use of health care services, lost days from work, unemployment, decreased quality of life, and premature mortality. Acute complications can also result in lost days from school. The total cost of diabetes in the United States in 2007 was $174 billion.

Despite its multi-system effects, it is possible to prevent or delay the onset of type 2 diabetes as well as to effectively manage both type 1 and type 2. Unequivocal evidence shows that early detection and early and aggressive ongoing therapeutic intervention significantly reduces the enormous human and economic toll from diabetes. To achieve the health benefits that modern science has made possible, the principal clinical features of diabetes—hyperglycemia, dyslipidemia, and hypertension—need to be prevented and managed within a system that provides continuous, proactive, planned, patient-centered, and population-based care. Primary care physicians, physician assistants, and nurse practitioners all play important roles in the delivery of primary care for people with chronic diseases in the United States. To reduce the risk of microvascular complications, this care needs to include regular assessment of the eyes, kidneys, teeth and mouth, and lower extremities in people with diabetes. System constraints, however, can make it difficult for primary care providers to carry out all of these essential elements of comprehensive diabetes care.

The challenge is to broaden delivery of care by expanding the health care team to include several types of health care professionals. Team care can minimize patients' health risks by assessment, intervention, and surveillance to identify problems early and initiate timely treatment. Increased use of effective behavioral interventions to lower the risk of diabetes and treatments to improve glycemic control and cardiovascular risk profiles can prevent or delay progression to kidney failure, vision loss, nerve damage, lower-extremity amputation, and cardiovascular disease. Patients' participation in treatment decisions, personal selection of behavioral goals, patient education and training, and active self-management can improve diabetes control. This in turn leads to increased patient satisfaction with care, better quality of life, improved health outcomes, and ultimately, lower health care costs.

Collaborative teams vary according to patients' needs, patient load, organizational constraints, resources, clinical setting, geographic location, and professional skills. It is essential that a key person coordinate the team effort. The resources and support of community partners such as school nurses, community health workers, trained peer leaders, and others can augment clinical care teams. Non-traditional approaches to health care such as telehealth, shared medical appointments, and group education all expand access to team care and, if used effectively, can build team care practices.

The benefits of diabetes team care include efficient patient education, improved glycemic control, increased patient follow-up, higher patient satisfaction, lower risk for the complications of diabetes, improved quality of life, reduced hospitalizations, and decreased health care costs. It is difficult, however, to measure team care effects beyond these intermediate outcomes. Future evaluations of model medical home health care delivery programs will likely provide additional data about improved patient outcomes.

Effective team care requires
- the commitment and support of organization leadership
- the active participation of the patient and health care professional team members
- ways to identify the patient population via an information tracking system
- adequate resources
- payment mechanisms for team care services
- a coordinated communication system
- documentation and evaluation of outcomes and adjustment of services as necessary

Teams can work effectively in many varied settings to improve the quality and effectiveness of diabetes care. Payment of services provided by health care professionals other than primary care providers and specialists—such as registered nurses, registered dietitians, and psychologists—although improving, often is inadequate. Examples in this guide from the peer-reviewed literature and case studies show the diversity and effectiveness of health care professional teams working with people with diabetes. These include
- community-based primary care providers who involve a pharmacist and dietitian in implementing treatment algorithms, nurse and dietitian case managers, and educators who help to improve patients' weight loss and A1C values
- a nurse practitioner-physician team that manages patients with diabetes and hypertension
- nurse and dietitian diabetes educators who help people with and at risk for diabetes achieve behavior-change goals leading to better clinical outcomes and who work with primary care physicians and staff to

provide "diabetes day" individual and group patient appointments
- school nurses who contribute to diabetes prevention and management in their students
- a nurse, social worker, or psychologist who works closely with older patients, their primary care physician, and a consulting psychiatrist to treat depression
- health care professionals who use telehealth to improve eye care, nutrition counseling, and diabetes self-management education
- pharmacists who work with company employees who have diabetes and their physicians to improve clinical measures and lower health care costs
- trained community-based fitness instructors who deliver group-based lifestyle interventions in YMCA settings to people at risk for diabetes to achieve increases in physical activity and significant weight loss
- trained community health workers who bridge the gap between traditional health care teams to improve access to diabetes health care, complications assessment, and education in underserved communities
- podiatrists and other health care professionals who help reduce lower-extremity amputation rates in foot care clinics
- dental and eye care professionals who help prevent and manage diabetes complications

There is evidence that a team approach reduces risk factors for type 2 diabetes, can improve diabetes management, and can lower the risk for chronic diabetes complications. This evidence, in turn, shows that an opportunity exists for health care professionals and health organizations to improve the health of people with diabetes. It is important, however, that studies of team care interventions involving the skills of numerous health care professionals should continue to elucidate effective ways to implement team care to improve patients' well-being and assess the costs involved.

For Team Care-Related resources see page 37.

1. Introduction

The problem

Diabetes is a serious, common, and costly chronic disease that affects 25.8 million Americans, or 8.3 percent of the U.S. population. About 1.9 million new cases are diagnosed annually.[1] Diabetes disproportionately affects African Americans, Hispanic Americans, American Indians, Asian and Pacific Islanders, and older Americans. Complications from the disease include cardiovascular disease, vision loss, kidney failure, nerve damage, and lower-extremity amputations. These complications can subsequently result in higher rates of disability, increases in the use of health care services, lost days from work, unemployment, illness, and premature death.

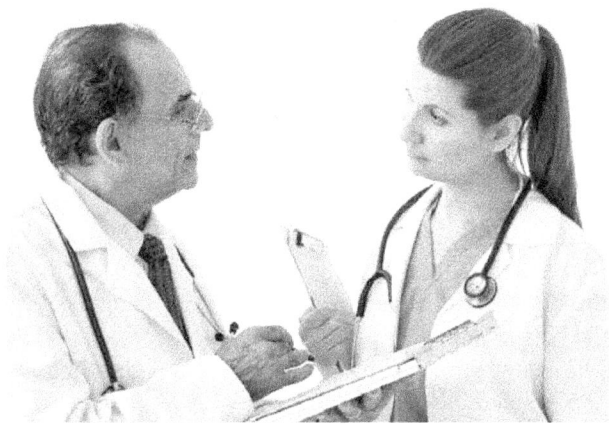

Type 1 and type 2 diabetes

Type 1 diabetes usually strikes children and young adults, although disease onset can occur at any age. In adults, type 1 diabetes accounts for 5 to 10 percent of all diagnosed cases of diabetes.[1] About 90 to 95 percent of people with diabetes have type 2 diabetes, which more commonly occurs in adults older than age 45 who are obese and have a family history of the disease. Overweight and obese children are at increased risk for developing type 2 diabetes during adolescence and later in life, with approximately one in three cases of new onset diabetes being type 2 in youths younger than age 18. This increased incidence of type 2 diabetes in youths is a first consequence of the obesity epidemic among young people and a significant and growing public health problem.[2]

Intensive versus standard therapy

Investigators in the Diabetes Control and Complications Trial (DCCT), a large clinical trial of intensive versus standard therapy for adults with type 1 diabetes, reported in 1993 that intensive glucose control reduced eye, nerve, and kidney damage. Findings reported in 2005 from the Epidemiology of Diabetes Interventions and Complications[3] (DCCT follow-up) study and in 2008 from the 10-year follow-up of the United Kingdom Prospective Diabetes Study (UKPDS)[4], show that intensive glucose control (A1C* goal <7 percent) in newly diagnosed people with either type of diabetes not only has benefits during the period of intensive therapy but also has a "legacy effect" in which micro- and macrovascular benefits are realized years later.

Cost of diabetes

The total cost of diabetes in the United States in 2007 was $174 billion, including $116 billion for direct medical costs and $58 billion in indirect costs, such as disability, time lost from work, and premature death.[5] Of the direct costs, 50 percent were for hospital inpatient care, 12 percent for diabetes medications and supplies, 11 percent for prescriptions to treat complications of diabetes, and 9 percent for physician office visits.

Computer modeling has shown that compared to standard treatment, early, effective diabetes management can reduce treatment costs for diabetes complications of the eye, kidney, and extremities.[6] There is a marked correlation between glycemic control and the cost of medical care, with medical charges increasing significantly for every 1 percent increase in A1C above 7 percent.[7] The increase in medical charges accelerates as the A1C value increases.

Prevention or delay of diabetes onset

About 79 million American adults have prediabetes and are likely to develop type 2 diabetes within 10 years, unless they take steps to prevent or delay diabetes.

Prediabetes occurs when a person's blood glucose is higher than normal but not high enough for a diagnosis of diabetes. The Diabetes Prevention Program (DPP), a large prevention study of people at high risk for diabetes, showed in 2002 that lifestyle intervention reduced the incidence of diabetes by an average of 58 percent over 3 years (by 71 percent among adults age 60 or older); diabetes incidence was reduced by 31 percent in those taking metformin.[8] A cost-effectiveness model estimated in 2005 that the DPP lifestyle intervention would cost society about $8,800 per quality-adjusted life-year saved (within a typically acceptable range). Metformin would cost about $29,900 per quality-adjusted life-year saved and was considered not cost-effective after age 65.[9]

In 2009, a 10-year follow-up of DPP participants, the Diabetes Prevention Program Outcomes Study, found that diabetes incidence was reduced by 34 percent in the lifestyle group and 18 percent in the metformin group compared with placebo. These results show that prevention or delay of diabetes with lifestyle intervention or metformin can persist for at least 10 years. [10] Interventions to prevent or delay type 2 diabetes in people with prediabetes are feasible and could be cost-effective.

Models for better diabetes care

The Chronic Care model,[11, 12] the Medical Home model,[13] and the Healthy Learner model[14] provide frameworks for effective care of diabetes and other chronic diseases. All incorporate team care as a vital component of delivery system design. These models will likely guide health care reform initiatives that incorporate an integrated health care delivery system.

This publication, *Redesigning the Health Care Team: Diabetes Prevention and Lifetime Management,* provides the following
- an overview of the evidence that supports team care as a component of effective diabetes management
- practical information to help health care professionals and organizations incorporate team care into practice in a variety of settings
- steps for forming and maintaining a successful team
- eight case studies that demonstrate real-world team care in several different settings

---

* NDEP and its partners have adopted the simple name "A1C" for the hemoglobin A1C test. A1C is a standardized blood test that indicates the average blood glucose over the previous 8 to 12 weeks. A1C values and self-monitoring of blood glucose can be used to guide therapy to achieve glycemic targets. People with diabetes need to know their own A1C values and whether they are reaching their targets.

For Team Care-Related resources see page 37.

2. Chronic Disease and the Health Care Delivery System

Health care environment

Today's health care environment is affected by several significant factors, including greater numbers of aging and older people, the development of new technologies, advances in medical treatments, and the tremendous increase in scientific knowledge about health and illness. One result is that more people are living longer with diabetes and its complications. In spite of the growing diabetes population and the high cost of this disease, people with diabetes are often poorly served by the current health care system that is primarily symptom oriented and focused on acute illness. Additionally, payment is heavily weighted toward medical procedures or treatment of late complications of disease, rather than toward the cognitive and time-consuming efforts required for successful primary or secondary disease prevention. Current payment policies need modification to support team care for effective chronic disease management.

Primary care providers

Primary care physicians, physician assistants (PAs), and nurse practitioners (NPs) all play important roles in the delivery of primary care for people with chronic diseases in the United States. Although endocrinologists or other diabetes specialty physicians are involved in caring for many people with diabetes, primary care physicians provide more than 80 percent of diabetes care.[15] In the past, physician shortages in rural or other underserved communities were addressed in part by PAs and NPs. Currently, however, about 33 percent of PAs practice in primary care, 15 percent practice in rural areas, and 8 percent in federally qualified health centers and community health facilities.[16] The PA profession appears to be moving away from primary care toward specialty training to support specialty physician practices. [17] NPs have traditionally worked in primary care, and a recent national survey reported that the average NP was female (95 percent), 48 years old, in practice for 10.5 years, and a family NP (49 percent) involved in direct patient care.[18] Schools of nursing are increasing training programs for doctoral-level comprehensive care practitioners.[17]

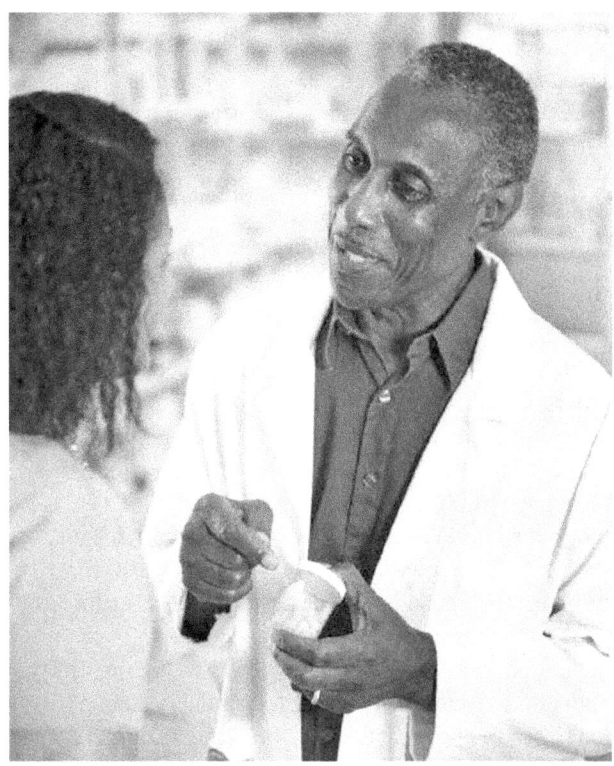

Systems constraints can make it difficult for primary care providers to carry out elements of comprehensive diabetes care, such as to
- identify a practice's sub-population of patients with diabetes and target those at highest risk for co-morbidities
- conduct ongoing self-management education and behavioral interventions
- provide remote management of glycemia
- promote risk-factor reduction and healthy lifestyles
- provide periodic examinations for early signs of complications[19]

The challenge is to broaden the delivery of primary care by expanding the health care team to effectively address the various elements of comprehensive diabetes care.

Models for care delivery

The models briefly described on the next page share many similar elements. Each element, however, is a complex undertaking, and the level of guidance available varies in its implementation and evaluation of effectiveness for improving chronic care.

Chronic care model

The chronic care model[11] presents six interrelated elements for effective care of chronic diseases:
- the health system–culture, organizations, and mechanisms to promote safe, high-quality care
- delivery system design–for clinical care and self-management support, including team care
- decision support–based on evidence and patients' preferences
- clinical information systems–to organize patient and population data
- self-management support–to enable patients to manage their health and health care
- community involvement–to mobilize patient resources

In 2002, a systematic review included diabetes care programs that featured at least one of four chronic care model elements: delivery system design, decision support, clinical information systems, and self-management support.[20] This review found that 32 of 39 programs improved at least one process measure (e.g., testing A1C) or one outcome measure (e.g., lowering A1C) for patients with diabetes by implementing at least one of the four chronic care model elements. Since the methodological quality of the studies was not uniformly high and the interventions differed among studies, the review authors cautioned about generalizing these findings.

In 2005, a meta-analysis[21] was conducted of randomized and non-randomized controlled trials in chronic disease that addressed one or more elements of the chronic care model. Diabetes was one of the four chronic diseases studied. This analysis found that interventions that incorporated at least one element of the model had consistently beneficial effects on process and outcome measures across the four diseases. Interventions for diabetes led to a 0.3-0.47 percent reduction in A1C but no measurable benefit in quality of life. The elements responsible for these benefits could not be determined from the data.

Medical home model

The American Academy of Pediatrics originally used the term "medical home" to describe a partnership approach to providing family-centered, comprehensive health care.[22] The model has since been embraced by the major U.S. primary care organizations, other health care provider groups, private health care purchasers, labor

unions, and consumer organizations. This evolving model of care is playing an important part in health care reform. [23]

Also known by other names such as the Advanced Primary Care model, the medical home links multiple points of health delivery by utilizing a team approach with the patient at the center. The model emphasizes prevention, health information technology, coordination of care, and shared decision making among patients and their health care team.[24]

Nurses, diabetes educators, dietitians, pharmacists, podiatrists, eye care providers, dental professionals, and other health care professionals are likely to play important roles in the medical home model by working with primary care providers to collaboratively provide comprehensive diabetes care. Such care includes management of blood glucose, lipids, and blood pressure; weight management; smoking cessation counseling; and diabetes complication care and prevention. Implementation of the medical home model will require modification of current health care provider payment policies to support team care.[25]

Medical home demonstration projects for Medicare beneficiaries are planned for community health centers across the country and for primary care practices in eight states. Medicare may join Medicaid and private insurers to conduct state-based primary care initiatives. These projects will incorporate payment modification for team care and evaluate the effectiveness of the model in improving health care quality and reducing costs.[24] Their findings will help guide future efforts to integrate and disseminate the model's key components, including payment mechanisms into other settings.[13]

Healthy learner model

The Healthy Learner Model extends the Chronic Care Model to include professional school nurses in chronic disease management for students in kindergarten through grade 12.[14] This model enables improved communication and coordination among health care professionals, students with chronic diseases and their families, and school personnel. The goal is to maintain student health in the school setting. Leadership involving communities and school districts is critical to the model as is evaluation of success in maintaining student health. The Healthy Learner Model has been successfully implemented and evaluated in Minneapolis Public Schools and St. Paul Public Schools to improve the health of children with asthma.[26] The model needs further application to diabetes and replication in other school districts.

3. What Makes a Successful Team?

Integral role of the patient and family

Team care integrates the skills of primary care providers and other health care professionals with those of the patient and family members into a comprehensive lifetime diabetes management program[19, 27] that is of high quality and is cost-neutral[28] or cost-effective. [29] The patient is the central team member, since most diabetes care is carried out by the person with diabetes or his or her family. Patients need to understand their roles as self-care managers and decision-makers to effectively work with members of their health care team. Family members assume most of this role for children and teens with diabetes.

Health care professionals

Teams usually include health care professionals with complementary skills who are committed to a common goal and approach.[30] Some health care professionals may choose to become certified diabetes educators (CDEs). (See Appendix 2 for information on the role of CDEs.)

Team composition varies according to patients' needs, patient load, organizational constraints, resources, clinical setting, geographic location, and professional skills. [31] It is essential that a key person coordinate the team effort. Non-traditional approaches to health care such as telehealth, shared medical appointments, and group education all expand access to team care.

What can team care accomplish?

Many examples of team management for people with diabetes can be found in the scientific literature. A 2006 meta-analysis assessed the impact on glycemic control of 11 distinct strategies for quality improvement in adults with type 2 diabetes.[32] Across 66 trials (50 randomized, three quazi-randomized, and 13 controlled before-after trials), two of 11 categories of quality improvement strategies were associated with reductions in A1C values of at least 0.5 percent. The two categories were team changes and case management.

- Effective team changes included the use of multidisciplinary teams, shared care between specialists

---

A flexible plan helps meet specific needs

Not every team member needs to be involved in every patient's care. A flexible plan helps determine the most effective team, as needs will change over time. For example

- A podiatrist may be involved in care for people with neuropathy, ulcerations, and other foot pathology. Podiatrists can provide comprehensive annual diabetes foot care examinations.
- A pharmacist may assist patients with multiple co-morbidities, or those requiring polypharmacy.
- Nurse educators, diabetes educators, and case managers can provide initial and ongoing diabetes self-management education, diabetes management support, and medication management services.
- Eye care professionals (optometrists and ophthalmologists) can provide comprehensive eye and vision care, including an annual dilated eye exam.
- A psychologist or social worker may be part of a team providing child and adolescent care.
- Dental professionals conduct oral examinations and provide oral health education in some community health centers.
- Clinical care teams can be augmented by the support and resources of school nurses, home health nurses, community health workers, and other community partners.

---

and primary care physicians, or adding a new team member with an expanded professional role.
- Effective case management involved nurse or pharmacist case managers who followed physician-supervised algorithms to make medication adjustments.

Similar results were found in a group of low-income Latino patients who received supervised, nurse-directed care using detailed treatment algorithms.[33]

Multidisciplinary teams are involved in pediatric care to effectively manage youths with diabetes.[34, 35] Team care contributed to the Steno-2 Study[36], a target-driven, long-term, intensified intervention that significantly reduced the risk of cardiovascular disease and microvascular events in adults with type 2 diabetes and microalbuminuria.[37] Although team care may have played a role in the success of other large clinical trials, there is little discussion of its contribution in the literature.

Possible Diabetes Team Care Outcomes

Studies of diabetes team care in a variety of settings (see section 6) have shown improvements in one or more of the following
- glycemic, lipid, and blood pressure control
- patient follow-up
- patient satisfaction
- risk for diabetes complications
- quality of life
- health care costs

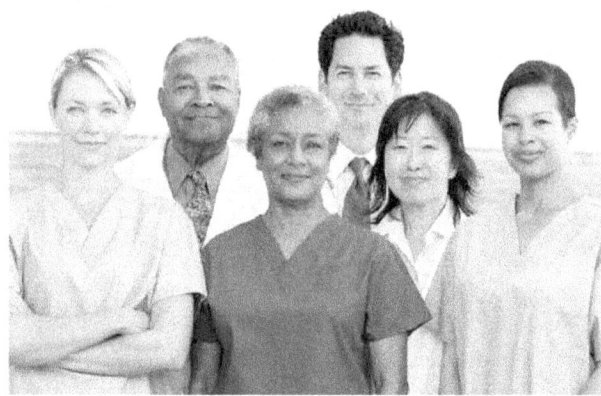

How to build and maintain effective teams

Six Team-building Steps presents important considerations for those creating or expanding team care, regardless of setting or program size: commitment of leadership; contributing team members; an identifiable patient population; adequate resources; a system for coordinated, continuous high-quality care; and an effectiveness evaluation plan.

Five Steps to Maintain a Successful Team presents elements that ongoing successful teams can promote: team coordination and communication; patient satisfaction, quality of life, and self-management; a community support network; patient follow-up; and the use of secure computerized clinical information systems.

Six Team-building Steps

These six steps identify important considerations for those creating or expanding team care, regardless of setting or program size.

1. Ensure the commitment of leadership

The first step requires care providers and other key decision-makers to commit to the implementation of multidisciplinary team care and the necessary resources and infrastructure to enable the team to function. A planning group can then carry out the next steps.

☐ Select well-respected clinicians to serve as catalysts to generate interest and support among colleagues.

☐ Meet with primary care providers and other potential team members, policy makers, and payment specialists such as business or office managers to obtain their support.

☐ Involve core team members early in organizational and clinical decision-making to gain their active participation.

☐ Demonstrate team care on a small scale, if necessary, to assess its feasibility, effectiveness, and impact.

2. Identify team members

☐ Invite potential team members to commit to participation.

☐ Clarify the roles of team members to resolve issues related to leadership and role overlap or redundancy in the care delivery process.[38]

☐ Ensure mutual respect and a common vision.

3. Identify the patient population

☐ Initial assessment may be limited to general demographic characteristics and an estimate of the proportion of patients with type 1, type 2, and gestational diabetes.

☐ Further assessment could determine the presence of risk factors, number of patients with and without diabetes complications, severity of complications, the extent of comorbidities, use of health services, and delivery of preventive care.[39]

☐ Once the diabetes patient population is known, the team might want to stratify the population into groups according to the intensity of services required.

  • Newly diagnosed patients with limited diabetes complications might benefit from relatively low-cost preventive care focused on risk factor reduction and health promotion.

  • Patients with diabetes complications or other comorbidities over the previous two-year period might need more intensive management with more extensive resources (see Appendix 1, Stratifying Team Care According to Patient Population Needs).

4. Assess resources

☐ Identify strengths and weaknesses in available resources (such as support staff, education materials, equipment, supplies, home care services, support groups, follow-up services, community resources). Ensure that adequate space, equipment, and supplies are available.

☐ Determine payment mechanisms for health care professional services, equipment, and supplies.

☐ Assemble user-friendly, current diabetes prevention and management protocols, tools, and education materials to ensure the delivery of current, culturally sensitive, and consistent care. These include standards of care, treatment guidelines, protocols and algorithms, patient education materials, flowcharts, standing orders, chart stickers, and other recording and reminder systems (see various resources in Resources section).

5. Develop a system for coordinated, continuous, high-quality care

☐ Define the team philosophy, goals, and objectives.

☐ Develop a secure information system for patient identification, data collection, ongoing assessment, and monitoring the achievement of specific clinical performance measures such as hemoglobin A1C, blood pressure, and lipid target values, as well as patient satisfaction and quality-of-life indicators.

☐ Determine the structure and scope of the program or service. Teams can provide medical and clinical care; diabetes risk-reduction counseling; diabetes, lipid, and hypertension management; self-management education and medical nutrition therapy; psychosocial counseling; complications risk-factor reduction counseling; screening for complications; follow-up care; coordination of referrals to specialists; and access to supportive clinical and community resources.

☐ Base care on evidence-based guidelines adapted from widely accepted standards or practice guidelines to meet local conditions.[40] (See various resources in Resources section.) Develop a system that supports continuity of care through regular team meetings and ongoing documentation and communication of pertinent information among team members, ideally via a computerized information system.

☐ Structure a payment system for professional services (see Resources–AADE, ADietA, CMS).

6. Evaluate outcomes and adjust as necessary

Periodic process and outcome evaluations can help to improve team function and patient care.

☐ Databases with analytic reports, pooled medical record audit findings, utilization data (such as hospital length-of-stay, emergency room visits, and total dollars spent) can help evaluate outcomes of team care, determine future progress, and indicate team success in meeting quality measures (see Appendix 3, Quality Improvement Indicators for Diabetes Care).

☐ Patient satisfaction and quality-of-life interviews or questionnaires for patients can provide valuable feedback to the team and may influence the scope and manner of care provided.

☐ Document clinical, behavioral, and financial outcomes to show payers and other stakeholders the value of the services and return on investment.

☐ If desired, teams could seek funding and resources from a nearby university or other facility for an evaluation expert for advice or to conduct a more formal program evaluation.

Five Steps to Maintain a Successful Team

Regardless of the team structure and purpose, several important elements need attention for ongoing, successful team care. These elements are presented below in no particular order.

1. Promote patient satisfaction, quality of life, and self-management

☐ Address patients' concerns such as insurance coverage and billing, confidentiality, time spent waiting, accessibility of providers, and continuity of care, to improve patient satisfaction.

☐ Provide self-management education to equip patients with the knowledge and skills to actively participate in their care, make informed decisions, set collaborative goals, carry out daily management, evaluate treatment outcomes, and communicate effectively with the health care team.

☐ Reassess and redefine collaborative goals and supportive care to sustain achievement of goals over time.

2. Promote a community support network

The support of family, friends, and the entire community can help people with diabetes sustain self-management practices and a positive outlook over time.

☐ Assess community support and resources such as institutional funding and grants from community agencies, groups, or services. Grants or industry support for indigent programs may be available.

☐ Determine available Medicare and other insurer payment for health care professional provider services (including diabetes patient education and nutrition counseling), equipment, and supplies (see CMS Resources).

☐ Help people with diabetes develop a community support network that includes family, friends, support groups, the faith community, and needed services such as transportation.

☐ Encourage community organizations to support routine physical activity and the concept of healthy foods for all to create an environment that can contribute to improved health outcomes and quality of life.

3. Maintain team coordination and communication

☐ Develop clear procedures to facilitate timely coordination of all required services.

☐ Consider using standard treatment algorithms (see various items in Resources).

☐ Reassess periodically to ensure continuity of care and patient satisfaction.

☐ Develop communication methods between team members and the patient such as team meetings, patient rounds, and journal clubs to promote cohesion and a common approach to patient care.

☐ Set individual patient clinical targets for blood glucose and lipid values, A1C, blood pressure, and body weight, and behavioral targets for food intake and physical activity. These targets provide a common ground for discussion of management strategies, collaborative goals, and evaluation of treatment outcomes.

☐ Develop and maintain consistent messages from all team members to enhance patient understanding and increase effective self-management behaviors.

☐ Communicate and document pertinent information from team members, ideally via a computerized information system.

☐ Encourage mutual respect between team members and the patient.

A multidisciplinary planning and documentation tool for the medical record could include treatment goals, personal patient goals, and disease management including medications, medical nutrition therapy, self-management education, and referrals. Such a tool can help all team members to clarify responsibilities, coordinate care, and communicate the patient's progress in a timely way.[38]

Referral reports from eye care, foot care, dental professionals, and others can be incorporated into the patient's health record through computer-generated reports, medical record notes, and personal and telephone contact. (See NDEP Resources for a microvascular checklist.)

4. Provide follow-up

Ongoing patient follow-up and regular scheduled visits for diabetes education, support, management, and preventive care are important to team success. A system to monitor and recall individuals for treatment and appointments, planned visits, and ongoing collaborative goal setting will facilitate the provision of these services.

- ❑ Essential preventive services include foot examinations; screening for microalbuminuria, visual acuity, and glaucoma; retinal eye examinations; and oral screening and preventive dental care.

- ❑ Follow-up care can be in the form of return face-to-face visits or interaction with other team members and community partners as well as telephone interviews and fax or email correspondence. Sending patients reminders and questionnaires encourages appointment keeping.

- ❑ Arranging for patients to send self-monitored data and to receive phone counseling and ongoing therapeutic management can reduce the need for multiple clinic or office visits, prevent adverse events, and increase access to care for patients in medically underserved locations.[41-43]

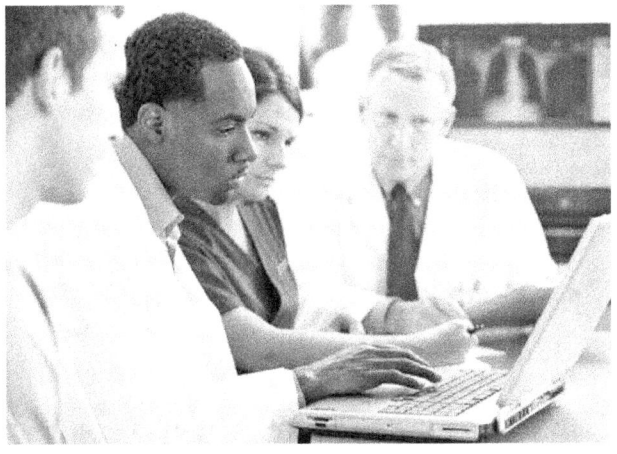

5. Use health information technology

Secure computerized clinical information systems can

- ❑ identify patients with diabetes, centralize their data and laboratory values, suggest a change in medication dosage, and enable timely referrals to other providers or specialists

- ❑ automatically remind the team to conduct self-management education, provide preventive services, and schedule follow-up visits

- ❑ help monitor quality of care by pooling medical record audit findings and comparing them with baseline measures or values attained in other practice settings

- ❑ collect and report outcomes

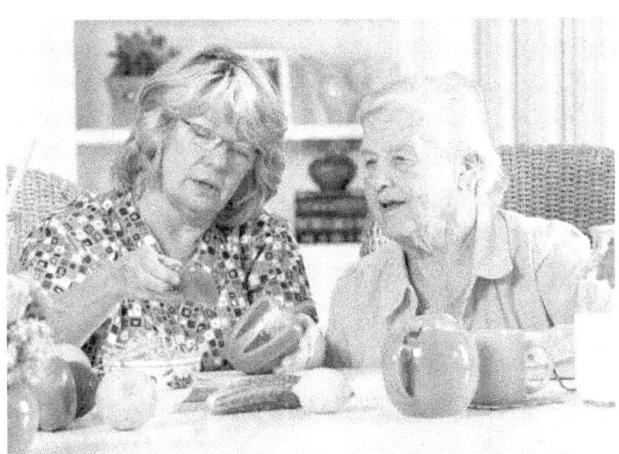

4. Non-traditional Team Care Approaches

Telehealth—Team care without walls

Telehealth applications

Telehealth (or telemedicine) is the use of secure high-speed Internet connections for real-time video conferencing for medical, diagnostic, monitoring, and therapeutic purposes when distance and/or time separates the participants. Telehealth can expand access to health care and education for patients and health care professionals in remote rural and medically underserved locations, as well as increase the delivery of evidenced-based medicine and improve the consistency of care.

Telehealth applications that expand the reach of the diabetes team include
- primary care digital retinal imaging for diabetes eye screening to augment or enhance regular comprehensive vision and eye health exams
- video conferencing for provider education (such as "Brown Bag" conferences)
- video conferencing for group diabetes education and individual counseling
- individualized telehealth for medical nutrition counseling (covered by Medicare)
- remote monitoring of self tests for blood glucose and blood pressure
- pediatric care for youth with type 1 diabetes in remote areas[44]
- shared web-based clinical information connecting the patient, endocrinologist, primary care provider, pediatric care experts, other specialists, and other team members
- secure email and remote management
- web-based patient surveys and information libraries
- customized patient portals or personal health records
- hospital "grand rounds" education sessions
(**See Case Studies 1 and 2** that address telehealth.)

Ocular telehealth programs

These programs can deliver eye care in the form of retinal screenings to those with limited care access and may in some cases improve care for those with regularly available vision and eye health care. Validated telemedicine programs using remote digital imaging systems are able to detect diabetic retinopathy but may not adequately detect other ocular co-morbidities associated with diabetes, including refractive errors, glaucoma, cataracts, dry eye, nerve palsies, and iris neovascularization. Retinal images are examined remotely by trained professionals.

The Indian Health Service (IHS)-Joslin Vision Network Teleophthalmology Program uses telemedicine technology to provide annual eye exams to American Indians and Alaska Natives with diabetes who live far from health care centers. A digital camera transmits photographs of a patient's eye to a central reading center, where IHS eye doctors interpret the images and send a report to the patient and primary care physician. The report includes the level of diabetic retinopathy, the presence of any non-diabetic retinal disease, and a recommended course of treatment. A four-year study showed that the program resulted in
- 50 percent increase in annual eye exams
- 51 percent increase in laser treatments to prevent blindness
- lower cost with quality equal to or better than a traditional dilated eye exam
(See IHS resources.)

Designing, building, and implementing an ocular telehealth program for diabetic retinopathy requires a clearly defined mission, goals (e.g., to preserve vision, reduce vision loss, and provide better access to limited forms of eye care), and guiding principles. When possible, these goals should be consistent with using telehealth to augment or enhance existing comprehensive eye care services. (See Resources under American Optometric Association and the Ocular Telehealth for two key documents that help an organization develop an effective and sustainable program.)

Early detection through annual screening and treatment of diabetic retinopathy can reduce vision loss by 90 percent.[45] Remote assessment of diabetic retinopathy using telemedicine is an accurate and potentially low-cost way to identify retinal lesions and facilitate appropriate and timely use of specialty care. Future studies will hopefully provide cost-effectiveness data of this service.

Case Study 1: Telehealth Enhances Diabetes Team Care in Hawaii

Joe Humphry, M.D.

Setting

Ms. LK is a 54-year-old Hawaiian female living on the Hamakua Coast on the Island of Hawaii with her husband and daughter. She has had type 2 diabetes for 10 years and associated hypertension and hyperlipidemia. She is under the care of a primary care physician at the rural community health center, which is about 10 miles from her home.

Team members

Team members include the patient and her family, primary care physician, eye specialist, chronic care nurse, community health worker, librarian, endocrinologist, and pharmacist.

Services provided at the Community Health Center

Ms. LK received her annual retinal screening using the teleophthalmology non-mydriatic camera at the health center. She previously had limited access to eye care. The retinal images were read by the Hawaii Telephthalmology Imaging Center, and the report was electronically sent to her primary care physician.

Ms. LK received education about insulin use and administration, and hypoglycemia management from the chronic care nurse when insulin therapy became necessary.

Services provided by the Native Hawaiian Health System

To help manage her diabetes, Ms. LK enrolled in the Native Hawaiian Health System remote monitoring program. As part of the program, a community health worker visited Ms. LK at home and delivered a blue tooth-enabled blood glucose (BG) meter and blood pressure (BP) cuff for BG and BP monitoring, demonstrated how to transmit the BG and BP readings after each reading, and uploaded the BG readings to the web-based Chronic Disease Management Program. Shortly after the upload, Ms. LK received a text message from her health care team thanking her for enrolling in the monitoring program. The community health worker referred Ms. LK and her daughter to the local public library for training to access her online portal and view her personal health record. The program donated a computer to the library in exchange for the librarian training of patients and patients' use of the computer.

Other aspects of the Chronic Disease Management Program include an educational library, patient alerts, email consultation, nutritional survey and assessment, behavioral health risk survey, electronic health record interface with the community health center, remote home monitoring, and a complete care plan. The program also conducts medication reconciliation to ensure that the patient is taking only currently prescribed medications and dosages.

Communication

The secure web-based Chronic Disease Management Program enabled the patient and the community health worker to communicate with the community health center physician and chronic care nurse. Ms. LK uploaded BG and BP readings for their review and received their instructions for adjusting her medication doses.

The community health worker recorded the findings of her patient visits for the community health center physician and chronic care nurse to review and to convey further instructions as necessary. The patient and other team members also conducted secure email consultations with an endocrinologist located on the Island of Oahu. The community pharmacist who refilled Ms. LK's medications was able to help her understand why she needed insulin.

Insurance coverage

In the current traditional payment system, the e-health activities and the outreach worker's time are not covered. The Community Health Center and the Native Hawaiian Healthcare System are compensated for "enabling services," making the e-health system a covered service. In the future, coverage will be through the management fee for the Medical Home Model or covered through an Accountable Care Organization Model* with a single payment to a larger organization that has an integrated delivery system. Kaiser Permanente currently uses many of the components of this system to reduce cost and improve access.

Outcomes

Ms. LK's insulin was effectively adjusted, and she took her BP medication daily. Her improved BG and BP values were recognized by the web application, and she received supportive text messages recognizing her improved diabetes management. The community health worker visited her every two weeks. Ms. LK visited the community health center physician and chronic care nurse every three months. Between visits, they were in touch via email. As a result of the telehealth support, face-to-face visit time focused on reviewing and setting self-management goals and discussing the support she needed to achieve her goals. Ms. LK took more responsibility for her diabetes self-management. Her self-monitored BG, A1C, and BP values improved.

*The Accountable Care Organization Model encourages physicians and hospitals to integrate care by holding them jointly responsible for Medicare quality and costs.

Other telehealth programs

These programs provide a sample of possible uses of telehealth to expand the team care concept.

The Arizona Diabetes Virtual Center of Excellence (ADVICE) is a comprehensive program for diabetes prevention, assessment, and management, carried out via Arizona Telemedicine Program Network.[46] The ADVICE program primarily provides diabetes education and individual telenutrition consultations in Spanish and English for Hispanics and American Indians who have inadequate access to health care.

The Indian Health Service is expanding its use of telemedicine to bring primary care and specialty medicine to remote locations to reduce geographic barriers between remote, smaller communities and health care professionals (see IHS resources).

Veterans Rural Health Resource Centers, opened by the Department of Veterans Health Administration in Vermont, Iowa, and Utah, are finding out how best to extend telehealth services to veterans living in rural areas (see Veterans Affairs Resources).

Case Study 2: Florida Initiative in Telehealth and Education for Children with Diabetes

Toree Malasanos, M.D.

This program was administered by the Florida Department of Health, Children's Medical Services Network (CMSN), to integrate telemedicine clinical care, web-based education for children with diabetes, and virtual home-based behavioral modification. The program has served about 99 children and their families (44 with diabetes and 55 with other endocrine disorders) in Volusia and Flagler Counties since 2001.

Targeted telemedicine patients were characterized by low socioeconomic status, inadequate health insurance, poor access to care, poor understanding of the diabetes disease process, transient lifestyles, residence in an area without access to a pediatric endocrinology specialist, and overall low health literacy. The program addressed several problems encountered in the pediatric endocrine and diabetes clinic:

- poor access to care for children with chronic health care needs in remote locations
- poor payment and minimal time for diabetes education
- high use of urgent care for recurrent problems rather than home management
- poor diabetes management and a high hospitalization rate

Services: Telemedicine clinical care

Patients were seen initially and then annually in person by the pediatric endocrinologist located in Gainesville, at the University of Florida. A teleconference clinic was held bi-weekly for an average of 12 families per session. Nurses in the remote clinic downloaded meter data, obtained a focused history, made basic physical observations, and transmitted the information to the endocrinologist in Gainesville. The pediatric endocrinologist then participated in patient interviews and examinations via real-time teleconferencing. Families were educated during the telemedicine visits and by the website about sick-day management and reasons to call the health care team. Families were supported in diabetes self-care by 24-hour telephone access to the endocrine team in Gainesville. Initial patient education was provided by a combination of "hands-on" education in Gainesville and the web education program. New guardians, families, teachers, and school nurses were invited to participate in the web education program, called Brainfood.

Services: Home-based behavior change

This statewide home-based virtual program replaced a model residential hospital unit with more than 20 years experience treating adolescents who had poor adherence, frequent hospitalizations, and impaired family dynamics. Families involved in the home-based program received three to five provider-initiated calls per week to encourage good diabetes self-management by addressing their individual barriers to care. Keys to the success of this program were a carefully designed curriculum based on the former residential program and provision of provider-initiated rather than family-initiated calls.

Web-based diabetes education (Brainfood)

This was an animated, multiple-literacy presentation of diabetes information (including material for non-readers), with pre- and post-testing. Children with newly diagnosed diabetes were given abbreviated in-person education at the University of Florida, which was then supplemented with Brainfood. Currently, this program is available at *www.myHealth-e.com*. It has been shown to increase knowledge about diabetes and its management.

Team members

Children with diabetes and their families worked as a team with the CMSN registered nurses, the pediatric endocrinologist, University of Florida registered nurses, a social worker and a nutritionist based at the remote clinic, and school nurses. A psychologist was part of the team for the home-based care. *Continued on next page.*

Florida has a state-funded telehealth program that provides diabetes care to pediatric patients who live in Daytona Beach and the surrounding areas and are insured through state and federal programs. At the time of a clinic visit, an on-site registered nurse obtains a standardized patient history, downloads the patient's blood glucose meter data, and faxes the information to the University of Florida, Gainesville, pediatric team. The nurse also arranges appointments with other providers such as a dietitian, a psychologist, or an ophthalmologist (**see Case Study 2**).

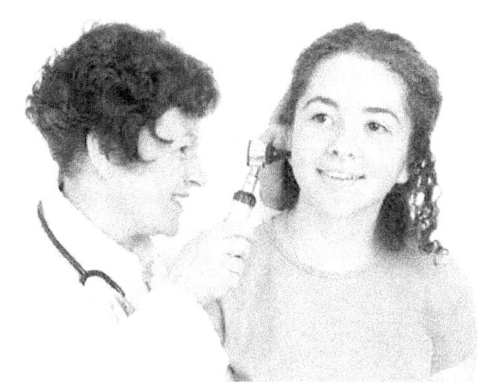

Case Study 2: Florida Initiative in Telehealth and Education for Children with Diabetes *Continued from page 16*

Payment for services

The program was funded by a contract with the Florida Department of Health, CMSN. Medicaid granted a waiver for limited coverage of telemedicine services for children with special health care needs in under-served regions of Florida. A contract between the University of Florida and the CMSN provided funds for data management and research, unreimbursed medical costs including physician time, phone management for blood glucose control between visits, and the home-based behavior-change program. This program was limited to CMSN and Medicaid clients; however, in states in which reimbursement for telemedicine services is allowed, private insurers typically follow the same pattern. (Medicaid reimbursement by state is described at *http://www.ichp. ufl.edu/documents/Telemedicine in Medicaid and Title V Report.pdf.*)

Outcomes

Hospitalizations and urgent care utilization: For the three years before inception of the program, there were on average, 13 hospitalizations per year (47 days) for the total group, which subsequently decreased by 88 percent to 3.5 hospitalizations per year (5.5 days) over the two years this was formally evaluated. Emergency department visits for the total group decreased from 8 per year to 2.5 per year. On numerous occasions, ketosis was managed by telephone intervention alone, relying on family-initiated calls.

Clinical measures: The mean interval between appointments was reduced from 149 days before the program began to 89–91 days over the two years this was formally evaluated. Of the children who had an A1C > 8 percent when they entered the program, the A1C dropped from a mean of 9.63 percent to 8.94 percent, p =.02. Of the chil-

dren who had an A1C less than 8 percent at their entry into the program, 100 percent stayed below 8 percent. After two years, the average A1C for all the children was 8.79 percent. Nineteen of 23 children received the recommended annual dilated eye examination.

Costs: Even when line charges and equipment of $18,826 were included, this program saved $27,860 per year, by reducing hospital days ($44,419/year) and emergency department visits ($2,267/year). This does not include transportation costs and work/school time saved. An additional savings of $64,978 could be considered if Medicaid transportation costs were included in the absence of the telemedicine clinic.

Satisfaction with the telemedicine clinic: A survey of the 99 program patients (diabetes, 44; other endocrine disorders, 55) and their parents found high levels of satisfaction with the program.

Related references

Bell JA, Patel B, Malasanos T: Knowledge improvement with web-based diabetes education program: Brainfood. Diabetes Technol Ther 2006; 8(4):4444–8.

Adkins JW, Storch EA, Lewin AB, et al.: Home-based behavioral health intervention: Use of a telehealth model to address poor adherence to type-1 diabetes medical regimens. Telemed J E Health 2006; 12(3):370–1.

Malasanos TH, Patel BD, Klein J, et al.: School nurse, family, and provider connectivity in the FITE diabetes project. Telemed Telecare 2005;11 Suppl 1:76–8.

Malasanos TH, Burlingame JB, Youngblade L, et al.: Improved access to subspecialist diabetes care by telemedicine: cost savings and care measures in the first two years of the FITE diabetes project. J Telemed Telecare 2005;11 Suppl 1:74–6.

Shared medical appointments and group education

A method to increase practice efficiency is shared medical appointments, where a multi-disciplinary team sees a group of patients. This model of care is a response to factors that include the increasing prevalence of chronic diseases such as obesity and diabetes, an aging population with a greater number of complex needs, the need to include family members in disease management and education, and limitations of the short traditional office visit.[47]

Structure and setting

Usually eight to ten patients participate every three months in a one- to two-hour appointment, although 20 or more patients can be seen in longer sessions.[48] Successful shared medical appointments for people with diabetes have been reported in various settings:
- health maintenance organizations[47, 49]
- a Veterans Health Administration (VHA) primary care clinic at a tertiary care academic medical center[48]
- a hospital-based secondary care diabetes unit[50]
- an adult primary care center serving uninsured or inadequately insured patients[51]

Interventions

Interventions usually focus on diabetes self-management support. Time is included for patients to meet individually with the primary care provider for evaluation of new medical problems, medication adjustments, and yearly checks for complications. Teams usually include two or more health care professionals, as needed, such as a family physician, clinical nurse specialist, nurse educator, NP, pharmacist, clinical health psychologist, dietitian, and podiatrist. Some of the health care professionals are certified diabetes educators (CDEs). Other care providers, such as eye specialists and dental professionals, could also be included. (See Appendix 2 for information on the role of CDEs.)

Evaluation

Success of the group visit model depends on
- skilled use of social and facilitation techniques by the health care team
- identification and scheduling of appropriate patients using a patient registry
- interpersonal sharing between patients
- training support staff
- active participation by all stakeholders[47]

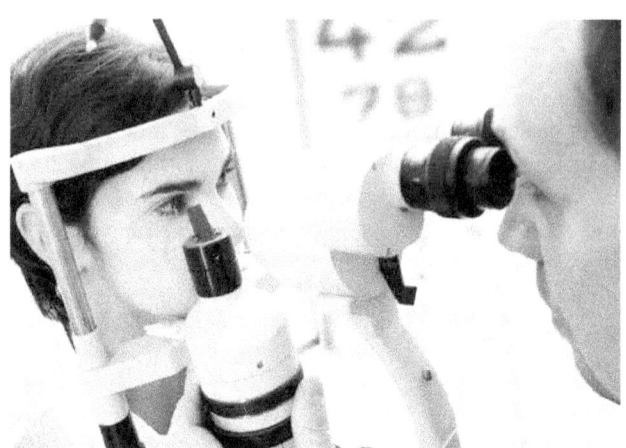

A meta-analysis of randomized controlled and controlled clinical studies of group education programs for adults with type 2 diabetes was compared with routine care, wait list control, or no intervention.[52] Studies were included if the intervention was at least one session with a minimum of six participants and if the length of follow-up was at least six months. Fourteen publications describing 11 studies that involved 1,532 participants were included. The analysis found significant improvements in
- fasting blood glucose levels and A1C
- self-care knowledge
- systolic blood pressure levels
- body weight

Diabetes medication dosage was reduced in one out of five participants.[52]

Other studies of group visits report
- fewer hospitalizations and emergency room visits[47, 49]
- improved quality of life[50]
- increased patient satisfaction[47]
- lowered cardiovascular risk [48]
- weight loss, smoking cessation, increased physical activity, and improved depression scores[53]

(**See Case Study 3** on group visits.)

Case Study 3: A Story about Group Visits

Michael Parchman, M.D.

Setting

A family physician in San Antonio considered why it was so hard for his patients to have optimal control of their A1C, BP, and cholesterol. He realized that he was trying to pack too much into each visit, and often spent 30–45 minutes providing patient education and support for some patients. He had previously worked in a community health center where group diabetes visits were offered, so he decided to conduct a group visit in his clinic.

Team members

The team included the physician and his office staff of two medical assistants, one licensed vocational nurse, three front desk staff, and one lab technician. A local representative from a pharmaceutical company was a certified diabetes educator and volunteered to teach a one-hour class during the group visit. The physician and team members held three planning meetings to prepare for the group visit. These meetings proved to be essential so that team members were prepared and understood their roles and responsibilities.

Services provided

The team selected a Friday morning three months in advance for the group visit. As patients with diabetes were seen in the clinic over the next three months, those with poor control of A1C, BP, or cholesterol were invited to attend the group clinic and were given an appointment for that Friday morning.

Each team member was assigned a "station" in each of three exam rooms where measures were obtained for A1C, LDL-cholesterol, and BP, respectively. The team member measured the required value and discussed the results with the patient. Each patient was given a station visit schedule, ending with a "medication station," where the physician reviewed the patient's medications; reviewed the patient's A1C, BP, and cholesterol values; and then made appropriate changes to the patient's medications if necessary.

After visiting all of the stations, the patients gathered in the reception area of the clinic for a one-hour discussion session with the diabetes educator. A healthy light lunch was provided.

Insurance coverage

A one-page template for documentation of the group visit was developed for billing purposes. Each staff member completed one portion of the template. The physician reviewed the documentation and completed the template during the one-on-one medication review with each patient. The visit with the doctor was billed using the usual CPT codes for primary care visits: 99213 or 99214.

Outcomes

Of the 20 patients invited, 17 attended. Interviews with the physician and office staff after the group visit revealed that the staff felt more involved in patient care and more satisfied with their role in the clinic than they had before the group visit. The physician felt more invigorated and was happier with his practice. Both the staff and physician reported improved patient understanding and improvements in patients' diet, physical activity, and medication-taking behaviors in the months following the group visit. Analysis of data from the charts before and after the group visits revealed declines in mean A1C from 8.5 to 8.0 percent; systolic BP from 142 to 132, and LDL-cholesterol from 124 to 99 mg/dl. Subsequent diabetes group visits were held every six months. The CDE pharmaceutical company representative continued to volunteer and teach a class during the group visits. The physician now also holds group clinic visits for patients with asthma.

5. Payment and Cost-Effectiveness Data for Diabetes Education and Services

Payment

One-on-one professional/patient services

Most health care plans pay for physician services provided for the management of diabetes. Medicare and many private insurance companies and managed care organizations pay for
- diabetes self-management education provided by an educator who is part of an accredited diabetes education program
- diabetes medical nutrition therapy (MNT) provided by a registered dietitian

Medicaid coverage for these services varies from state to state.

To receive payment for MNT services provided to a Medicare beneficiary with diabetes, a registered dietitian must be a Medicare provider and follow specific MNT payment rules written by the Centers for Medicare and Medicaid Services (CMS) (see Resources under CMS).

Self-management diabetes education program services

To receive Medicare payment for diabetes self-management education services, outpatient diabetes education programs must meet defined standards. There are currently two organizations that have the authority to accredit, or recognize, diabetes education programs:
- American Diabetes Association (ADA)
- American Association of Diabetes Educators (AADE)

(See Resources under ADA and AADE.)

Recognized diabetes education programs exist in a variety of settings, including hospital out-patient clinics, physician's offices, home care agencies, pharmacies, and community facilities.

Recognized programs need to meet all requirements developed by CMS for Medicare payment. Diabetes self-management education requires a G billing code for either individual or group education. (See Resources under CMS, AADE, and American Dietetic Association for information about Medicare diabetes self-management education and MNT payment provided in a variety of practice settings.)

Medicare-covered items

Medicare covers numerous tests, equipment, supplies, medications, and services for enrolled people with diabetes and those at risk of diabetes (see Appendix 4). To date, most states have passed legislation ensuring varying degrees of coverage for the above items for persons whose insurance plans are regulated by state law.

Billing practices and CPT codes

To maximize insurance coverage of team member contributions to the patients' care, it is important to know the billing practices in a local area and allowable fees and to use the correct CPT codes (see Resources under AACE, AADE and AAFP).

"Incident to" billing

"Incident to" billing can be applied to patients billed under Medicare's traditional fee-for-service system for services that are integral although incidental to the physician's personal professional services. Commercial payers and some private payers may use a similar billing procedure. The "incident to" rules (listed in the *Medicare Carriers Manual*) cover services rendered by other health care professionals when the services are
- supervised by the physician who is on site at the clinic or office at the time of service and who is actively involved in the patient's course of treatment
- furnished by a person who is an employee of the physician (there may be exemptions)
- documented clearly in the medical record

This billing procedure does not apply to MNT or to diabetes education services.

Cost-effectiveness evidence for diabetes education

Systematic reviews

Summaries of six systematic reviews of diabetes education and related costs emphasize that many studies did not include full economic analyses.[54-59] Education was provided in a variety of settings and included individual and group education by a variety of health care professionals. Although most of the studies indicated that diabetes education was likely to be cost-effective, a common conclusion of the reviews was that further research is needed, including full economic analyses and use of well-defined education programs that are reproducible.

Observational studies

Two more recent observational studies have concluded that diabetes education does result in reduced health care costs. One study of 18,404 patients with diabetes concluded that any type of diabetes educational visit (as opposed to none) was associated with 9.18 fewer hospitalizations per 100 person-years and $11,571 less in hospital charges per person.[60] Each visit to a nutritionist was associated with 4.7 fewer hospitalizations per 100 person-years and $6,503 less in hospital charges per person. Patients were included in the database if they had a diagnosis of diabetes recorded between March 1, 1993 and December 3, 2001 and at least a one-month follow-up period. The mean follow-up period was 4.7 years. Encounter-form data, including several types of education visits from a variety of health care professionals, were linked with hospital discharge data for the same period. Some diabetes educators were certified while others had either a relevant degree or relevant training and experience.

The second observational study reviewed 482,500 commercial and 152,000 Medicare claims in payer-derived complete three-year data sets for 2005 through 2007 that were linked with several codes for diabetes education services.[61] Commercially insured members and Medicare members who participated in diabetes education cost on average 5.7 percent and 14 percent less, respectively, than members with diabetes who did

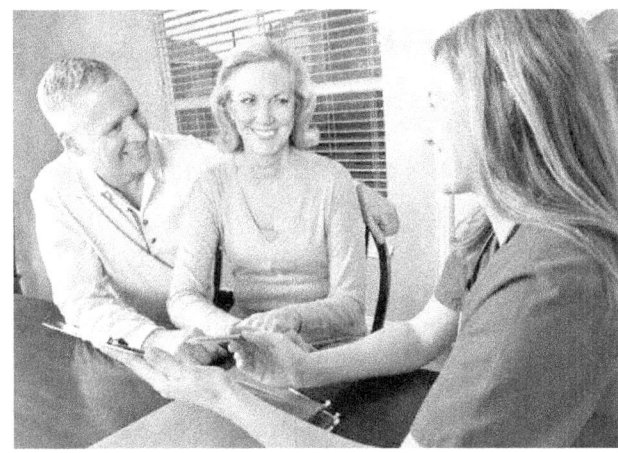

not participate in diabetes education. Diabetes education in the commercial group was associated with higher use of primary and preventive services and lower use of acute, inpatient hospital services. The gap in costs for the commercial population between the diabetes education and the non-education groups increased over time so that by year three, the non-education group average cost was 12 percent higher. A similar but smaller gap developed in the Medicare population's costs. Claims for Healthcare Effectiveness Data and Information Set (HEDIS) diabetes process measures were positively correlated with the prevalence of diabetes education at the provider practice level. Physician referral rates for diabetes education varied considerably.

The findings of both of these observational studies imply that participating in diabetes education is associated with improved clinical outcomes that, in these cases, related to fewer hospitalizations or lower overall health care costs.

Guide to develop a business case

A handbook produced by the Diabetes Initiative of the National Program Office at Washington University School of Medicine provides a guide for diabetes education programs to develop a business case for the cost-effectiveness of programs, which can be used with administrators and payers.[62]

6. Collaborative Care in Practice

These examples are a selection of relatively recent studies that, in combination, show the diversity of team care in practice. The studies measure different endpoints, and few measure improved patient morbidity. They do, however, provide practical examples of collaborative care for diabetes prevention and management in a variety of practice settings with different professional team members. The examples are categorized by practice setting and health care professional involvement—and are in alphabetical order.

Practice Setting

Community settings

Partnerships between health care professionals, community organizations, and community members may help widen the reach of diabetes prevention services for people at high risk for diabetes, as well as of diabetes management programs.

The Building Community Supports for Diabetes Care program of the Robert Wood Johnson Foundation Diabetes Initiative works through clinic-community partnerships. Several projects demonstrate how various clinic-community partnerships promote diabetes self-management better than any organization could do so alone. They are also real-world examples for the community involvement element of the chronic care model.[63]

Diabetes prevention in adults

In people at risk of developing diabetes with modifiable risk factors, low-cost, intensive lifestyle interventions delivered at YMCA facilities to modify eating and exercise behaviors have thus far shown promising results in reducing risk of diabetes. Trained community-based fitness instructors were able to deliver an effective group-based lifestyle intervention in YMCA settings to adults at high risk for diabetes.[64] Pilot studies suggest that participants achieved weight loss similar to that achieved in the original Diabetes Prevention Program. Significant changes included decreased body weight and total cholesterol maintained over 12 months.[65]

Diabetes prevention in children

A three-armed randomized controlled clinical trial used trained extension workers to lead group sessions over 16 weeks for 93 overweight or obese children ages 8 to 14 (who were at risk for diabetes) and their families. Families were randomized into a behavioral family-based intervention, a behavioral parent-only intervention, or a wait-list control group. At the 10-month follow-up, children in both intervention groups had significantly greater decreases in body weight compared with the control group.[66] A comparison of intervention costs showed that the total program costs for the parent-only and family interventions were $13,546 and $20,928, respectively. Total cost per child for the parent-only and family interventions were $521 and $872, respectively. The authors concluded that parent-only interventions may be cost-effective for pediatric obesity management, especially for families in medically underserved settings.[67]

Diabetes management

Connecting with community health workers

Trained community health workers are playing an increasingly important role in bridging the gap between traditional health care systems and needed diabetes health care and education in underserved communities. Through their understanding of a community's language, cultural beliefs and traditions, and barriers to care, community health workers can help health care professionals and their patients achieve more effective diabetes prevention and management and make better use of the health care system.[68]

(See AADE Resources for a position statement regarding the role of community health workers in diabetes care. See CDC Resources for a review of the capacities and contributions of community health workers; also **see Case Study 4.**)

Peer support

There is growing interest in the role of peers as providers of on-going diabetes self-management support. Peer support links people living with diabetes who are able to share knowledge and experiences. Peer support can take

Case Study 4: Using Community Health Workers to Improve Quality in Diabetes Care

Jon Liebman, M.S., M.S.N., and
Dawn Heffernan, M.S.N.

Setting

Holyoke Health Center (HHC) in Holyoke, Massachusetts, has two sites that serve about 20,000 patients, most of whom are Spanish speaking. More than 1,700 of the adult patients have diabetes. In 1999, HHC adopted an electronic registry to track these patients and their clinical data. In 2003, HHC began using the data registry to identify patients lost to routine follow-up or who were in poor glycemic control and at risk for adverse outcomes.

Team members

Team members included primary care providers, a primary nurse, a pharmacist, a diabetes educator, a nutritionist, and medical assistants. In 2003, trained community health workers were added to the diabetes care team to engage and support patients who were not succeeding in managing their diabetes.

Services

Adults in poor diabetes control were targeted by community health workers for phone outreach and, as needed, home visits, to assist them to reestablish primary medical care. The health workers functioned as a link between patients and their physician and other team members to help resolve problems and assist patients in overcoming barriers to implementing diabetes self-care behaviors.

Communication

In addition to team meetings and telephone contact, the team members communicated through formalized documentation tools in the medical record, including progress notes, in-house referrals, and shared Excel spreadsheets to outline the current services and community health worker assignments.

Insurance coverage

The initial project, Proyecto Vida Saludable, was funded by the Robert Wood Johnson Foundation. Other funders have included the Health Resources and Services Administration, Massachusetts Department of Public Health, Massachusetts Association for the Blind, Blue Cross Blue Shield, and Massachusetts Medical Society.

Outcomes

Improvement in two key indicators may partially reflect the effects of the interventions. First, the proportion of patients with diabetes who had been seen within the previous three years but who had not had an appointment within the previous year was reduced from 28 percent to 6.5 percent. Second, over three years, the average A1C was reduced from 8.4 percent to 7.5 percent, and the proportion of patients with an A1C >10 percent decreased from 18.2 percent to 10.8 percent.

Related reference

Liebman J, Hefferman D: Quality improvement in diabetes care using community health workers. Clinical Diabetes 2008; 26(3): 75-76.

---

many forms: phone calls, text messaging, group meetings, home visits, and shared activities. Peers can provide emotional, social, and practical assistance to help others manage their diabetes and stay healthy. Peers can help others with diabetes to

- figure out how to manage diabetes in their daily lives
- identify key resources for healthy foods or for physical activity
- cope with social or emotional barriers
- stay motivated to reach their goals
- seek out clinical care as appropriate
- stay engaged in diabetes self-care over the long term[69]

Receiving social support may contribute to self-efficacy, medication adherence, and improved self-reported health status. Peers who provide social support may experience less depression, heightened self-esteem and self-efficacy, and improved quality of life.[69] (See Resources under Peer Support.)

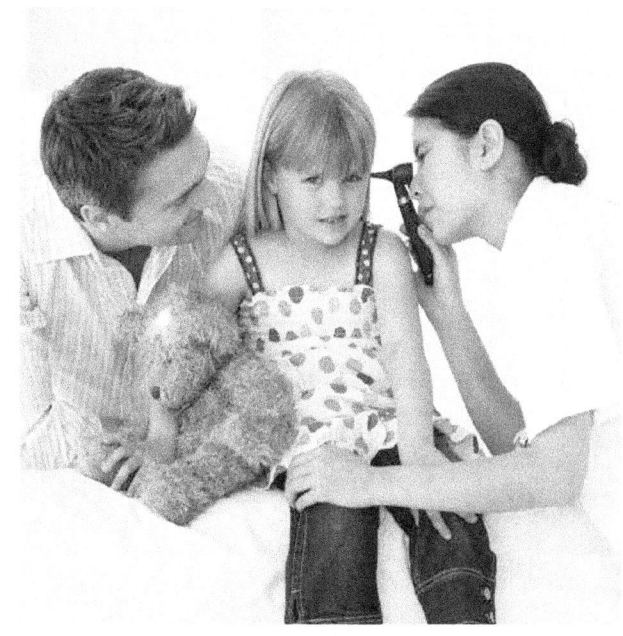

Managed care

A study of clinical outcomes in a large managed care population of adults with diabetes showed that compared to usual care, computer-supported care by a dedicated health care team appeared to reduce the number of hospitalizations and improve measurement rates for A1C, urinary protein, and serum lipid. Glycemic control and blood pressure control also improved.[70]

In a health maintenance organization's pediatric diabetes self-management program, a nurse case manager and a multidisciplinary clinic team provided education and counseling to empower families to improve their child's self-management of diabetes. The means of all measures of self-management improved, as did parents' self-efficacy beliefs.[71]

In Arizona, six competing, capitated Medicare managed care plans collaborated with a peer review organization to improve outpatient diabetes team management for their members. One year after baseline measures were taken, there was significant improvement in most indicators. Mean A1C values fell from 8.9 percent to 7.9 percent; the proportion of patients with A1C values <8 percent rose from 40 percent to 62 percent; the use of ACE inhibitors increased by 69 percent; and the treatment of dyslipidemia improved from 16 percent to 40 percent. There was no significant improvement in lipid profiles.[72] (**See Case Study 5** for an example of team care in a managed care setting.)

Multidisciplinary foot care clinics

A number of studies have reported that multidisciplinary foot care programs have successfully reduced lower-extremity amputation rates.[73-75] Coordination of activities between various disciplines involved in diabetes-related foot care—including surgeons, medical specialists, podiatrists, diabetes educators, and ortho-

---

Case Study 5: A Collaborative Team Approach to Managing Diabetes in a Clinic Setting

Roger P. Austin, M.S., R.Ph., C.D.E.

Setting

The Henry Ford Health System in Detroit, Michigan, operates four Diabetes Care Centers in outpatient clinic facilities geographically distributed across metropolitan Detroit.

Team members

Registered nurses, nurse practitioners, and clinical pharmacists who are also CDEs, primary care physician "champions," and specialty care physicians of the Henry Ford Medical Group.

Services

The Diabetes Care Centers' services require referral from a physician who is part of the closed medical group practice model. Any patient with diagnosed diabetes and an A1C >7 percent is eligible for referral. Clinic enrollment is intended for six months and involves frequent interaction with the patient via face-to-face visits, telephone, or email. Services include an initial assessment of the patient's major concerns about diabetes self-management and associated self-care behaviors (eating patterns, physical activity, medication taking, stress management, problem-solving ability, self-monitoring of blood glucose, and risk-reduction practices). Patients are screened for depression and possible referral for behavioral health counseling. Motivational interviewing methods help patients actively engage in their disease management. Referrals are made as necessary to other Henry Ford Medical Group specialists including cardiology, nephrology, neurology, ophthalmology, and podiatry.

A unique feature of the clinic services is limited, delegated, prescriptive authority to the CDE pharmacist "coaches" who manage and change the patients' medications using health system-approved treatment algorithms for management of hyperglycemia, dyslipidemia, and hypertension. This allows for rapid-cycle progression of therapy, as required, to help patients achieve therapeutic goals for blood glucose, lipid, and blood pressure. Coaches are authorized to order laboratory tests as necessary to help monitor patients' responses and to adjust medications.

Communication

All coach/patient encounters are documented in the electronic medical record system. All coach actions and notes require physician approval. Telephone and email contact enhance clinical decision-making.

Insurance coverage

Diabetes care services receive capitated coverage from the health system and certain preferred provider organizations.

Outcomes

Patient satisfaction feedback surveys that are sent to all diabetes center enrollees have been uniformly positive. The clinical study that evaluated the concept for this service showed a clinically significant decrease in A1C levels of nearly 1 percent in the study population (unpublished study).

tists—appears to be very important for lowering amputation rates.[76] (**See Case Study 8** for an example of team care in a foot care clinic.)

The Veterans Health Administration (VHA)

The VHA Prevention Amputation Care and Treatment Program (PACT) uses a multidisciplinary team approach to identify patients at risk for amputation, which include those with diabetes, end-stage renal disease, and peripheral vascular disease. Once identified, the program provides a mechanism to screen those "at-risk" veterans for foot risk factors in primary care clinics, and to provide timely and appropriate referral to specialists. The foot screening involves the

- use of the 10gm monofilament to screen for loss of protective sensation
- palpation of pedal pulses to screen for diminished arterial blood flow
- inspection for foot deformities that often lead to foot ulcers

The program uses a series of unique databases to provide ongoing performance measurements (amputation levels and rates and ulcer types and rates, as well as data on patient demographics and "at-risk" and "high-risk" foot conditions). PACT monitors continuity information about clinic visits to primary care and foot care clinics to identify those at highest risk who may require additional outreach efforts.

In 2008, the nationwide compliance with the screening performance measure for the monofilament testing for veterans with diabetes was 88 percent. The amputation rates for pcoplc with diabetes have declined from 8.5 per 1,000 in 2001 to 4.2 per 1,000 in 2008 (see Veterans Affairs Resources).

Primary care clinics

A small, rural primary care clinic that included a critical access hospital and a 25-provider physician group implemented care practices in 2006 that improved A1C values in all patients with type 2 diabetes. The clinic adopted practice guidelines with algorithms for care, and a pharmacist and dietitian provided diabetes self-management counseling. A diabetes flowchart was used to track care and a registry maintained relevant data.[77]

A pilot study with six primary care providers in a rural practice introduced a diabetes nurse educator to work with the physicians and their patients with diabetes. Results showed improvement in patients' knowledge and empowerment, and A1C and HDL values.[78]

Compared with care provided by the primary care physician alone, a nurse practitioner–physician team improved care to patients with hypertension and diabetes. In the team-treated group, one-year costs for personnel were modestly higher, but participants experienced significant improvements in mean A1C and HDL values and in satisfaction with care.[79] A primary care physician in a large multi-specialty medical group introduced team care to his practice and improved quality-of-care indicators for patients with diabetes.[80] (**See Case Study 6** for an example of team care in a primary care setting.)

Stepped diabetes management

In stepped care, the team assesses patients' management concerns, skills, and resources and then sets education and treatment goals in collaboration with patients. Precise timelines are set for success with individual therapies. The team provides different steps or levels of treatment according to predetermined protocols until management goals are met and maintained. Combined evaluation data are generated for providers to compare changes in practice with baseline measures. This approach was tentatively estimated to generate lifetime savings of about $27,000 per patient after six to seven years when modeled with the costs of acute and chronic complications.[81] More recently, in an academic family practice clinic, stepped care resulted in significant cost-neutral improvement in A1C values.[82]

Health Care Professional Involvement

Dental professional team members

Oral health care professionals play an important role as part of the health care team by providing oral care to patients with or at risk for diabetes. Glycemic control may exacerbate periodontal disease and, conversely, periodontal disease may cause deterioration of glycemic control. Growing evidence supports this bidirectional link between periodontal disease and diabetes, but further research is needed to understand this relationship. The IDF *Guideline on Oral Health for People with Diabetes* recommends that diabetes care providers incorporate oral health into diabetes education and refer patients to dental health professionals annually for oral health care.[83]

Few studies probe the financial impact of the periodontal disease-diabetes relationship. Some research indicates increased dental costs for people with diabetes.[84] Dentists and dental hygienists can work with the physician, diabetes educator, and dietitian to maintain the patient's oral health and possibly improve the patient's metabolic control of diabetes. New screening tools will enable dentists to detect and refer undiagnosed cases of diabetes.[85] Reducing tobacco use via anti-tobacco promotion and tobacco-cessation programs could improve both cardiovascular health and oral health.[86]

Depression care managers

Older patients with diabetes and depression who received team care via the IMPACT program (Improving Mood-Promoting Access to Collaborative Treatment for Late Life Depression) had an average of 115 more depression-free days, better physical functioning and quality of life, and lower medical costs over two years than did patients treated with standard care. The lower costs more than offset the cost of the team care. The IMPACT team includes a depression care manager (usually a nurse, social worker, or psychologist) who works closely with the patient's primary care physician and a consulting psychiatrist to treat depression in the patient's regular primary care clinic.[87, 88]

Eye care professionals

Achievement of the Healthy People 2010 objective to improve rates of preventive annual dilated eye examinations in people with diabetes was assessed in 59 CDC Diabetes Prevention and Control Programs. Results showed that from 2000 to 2003, the aggregate, age-adjusted rate of annual dilated eye examinations decreased from 67.7 percent to 65.2 percent (P=.05).[89] Ophthalmologists and optometrists are critical members of the health care team with unique responsibilities for diabetes eye health.[90] Implementing recommendations for annual dilated eye examinations is essential to help prevent vision loss from diabetic retinopathy.

Case Study 6: Clinica Family Health Services: Enhanced Team Functioning

Carolyn Shepherd, M.D.

Setting

The Clinica Family Health Services community health center provides care to a largely uninsured Hispanic population of about 40,000 patients at four sites near Denver, Colorado. The health center was one of the first to participate in the Health Disparities Collaborative of the federal Bureau of Primary Health Care and has worked to improve primary care practice since 1999. The center has made major organizational and cultural changes in the process of forming its high-functioning teams.

Team members

Primary care teams are called "pods." There are four pods at one site, two at another, and three pods at each of the two other sites. Each pod is color coded to help patients identify with their care team and to improve continuity of care—the walls and the primary care provider business cards and appointment cards are differently colored.

Each pod has three full-time equivalent primary care clinicians: physicians, NPs or PAs, and certified nurse midwives. Medical assistants usually work with a single clinician, contributing to continuity of care. Pods also have a nurse team manager, who is either a registered nurse (RN) or a licensed practical nurse (LPN). Pods share a referral case manager, social worker, office manager, and financial screener. The organization has a registered dietitian who is a CDE. The dietitian helps train RNs and LPNs, supports group visits for people with diabetes with their primary care provider, and counsels individual patients with diabetes. All clinicians and staff who care for patients are required to be bilingual Spanish speakers.

Services

To improve continuity of care, each of the 60 or more primary care clinicians has his or her own panel of 1,000 to 1,200 patients. This panel size maximizes the goal that patients see the same clinician whenever possible at each visit and has improved access to care. The primary care clinicians assess and manage current medical problems and comorbid conditions. For chronic diseases such as diabetes, computer-generated registries, reminders of checks for diabetes management, and status of complications help clinicians provide timely care.

The referral case managers, often high school graduates trained by the center, relieve clinicians of the time-consuming efforts to arrange appointments and negotiate payment for services. Pod case managers help patients set self-management goals, do brief screenings for depression, counsel patients with mild to moderate depression, and help with tobacco cessation follow-up and referrals.

Medical assistants take vital signs, document history of present illness, screen for tobacco use, room patients, draw blood, and do depression screens. Working with pod receptionists, they manage the chronic disease registries and order overdue tests. Up-to-date registry data are pulled directly from the electronic health record database and displayed, using crystal reports and business intelligence tools.

RNs and LPNs play a central role. They coordinate team activities, oversee the medical assistants, and provide health education. They activate diabetes patients to manage their illness by providing diabetes education and seeking patients' input for goal setting during each

Continued on next page.

Efforts to improve coordination among team members to facilitate referral for eye examinations can increase eye care in low-income, uninsured populations.[91] Multidisciplinary patient-centered vision care algorithms have been developed to help patients with diabetes to access appropriate screening and management of diabetic retinopathy.[92] A standard reporting form for eye examination results can be easily used in clinical practice[93] (see American Optometric Association resources). A comprehensive microvascular complications checklist is being developed by the NDEP.

Nurse and dietitian certified diabetes educators

A program to implement and financially sustain an effective diabetes self-management education program was implemented for patients seen in community hospitals and primary care practices in the western part of Pennsylvania.[94] Nurse and dietitian CDEs worked with primary care office staff to provide "diabetes day" individual and group patient appointments. Results showed increased patient access to these education services, improvement in A1C levels, and increased nurse involvement in medication initiation and adjustments, and patient satisfaction. Recognition from the American Diabetes Association in 21 sites enabled billing practices to help cover costs through payment for the educators' services (**see Case Study 7**).

Pharmacists

By taking nontraditional roles in family practice or medicine clinics in both urban and rural communities, pharmacists can improve chronic disease management,

---

Case Study 6: Clinica Family Health Services: Enhanced Team Functioning

Continued from page 26

visit. Patients choose their own self-care goals as part of their self-management plans. Lessons learned in self-management are then applied by the patient toward other health care goals such as walking or stopping tobacco use. Under a primary care provider's supervision, RNs and LPNs screen for and treat simple infections, obtain urine cultures, and contact patients.

Communication

Clinical sites are organized so that pod teams work in the same open room at the pod's center, from which they can see all the patient rooms. This enables team members to easily and quickly communicate with one another. Incoming calls are routed to a centralized call center. Calls with clinical content go to the pod receptionist, who also contacts patients with normal lab results, checks patients in and out of their visits, and helps manage chronic disease registries. Outgoing calls are generally made by the case manager, LPN, or medical assistant, using clinical protocols or specific instructions from the clinician to inform patients of abnormal lab results, schedule periodic care, schedule patients in group visits with their primary care provider, and refill prescriptions. Since most of the patients do not have health insurance, the clinic uses a digital retinal camera to screen patients and determine who needs to be referred for specialty eye care.

Insurance coverage

More than half of Clinica Family Health Services patients do not have any health insurance coverage. The cost of care to these patients is supported by a 330 Federally Qualified Health Center grant. Services to patients with diabetes are billed to state Medicaid and Medicare when the patient has this coverage. Less than eight percent of patients have private insurance.

Outcomes

Continuity of care with the patient's primary care clinician is 80 percent for well care, 70 percent for diabetes care, and 60 percent for acute care such as asthma visits. Access to care is three days or fewer for established patients compared to three weeks to three months prior to the formation of patient panels, and patients' no-show rate has dropped from 35 percent to eight percent.

A summary of Clinica Family Health Services's self-reported data showed that the average A1C level of its population (now 1,916 patients) with diabetes dropped from 10.5 percent in October 1998 to 7.9 percent in November 2009. The percentage of patients with diabetes with at least two A1C tests within a year rose from 11 percent in October 1998 to 92 percent in November 2009. The percentage of patients with diabetes self-management goals rose from three percent in February 1999 to 50 percent in November 2009. The percentage of those having foot examinations rose from 15 percent to 62 percent in the same period. Since 2007, these data have been pulled from the EMR database and now include 100 percent of the diabetes population for every measure.

Related references

Shepherd C: Clinica Family Health Services: Using space and financial incentives to enhance team functioning. In: Bodenheimer T, ed. Building Teams in Primary Care: 15 Case Studies. Oakland, CA.: California Health Care Foundation, 2007; 9-11.

Bodenheimer T, Wagner EH, Grumbach K: Improving primary care for patients with chronic illness. JAMA 2002; 288(14): 1775-9.

utilizing education and counseling skills or collaborative practice agreements with physicians.

Pharmacist interventions

A systematic review of 21 published studies of pharmacist interventions with adults with diabetes included nine randomized controlled trials, one controlled trial, and 11 cohort studies with a control group. Findings demonstrated consistent positive effects on patient A1C, lipids, and blood pressure values. Many pharmacist-based models were used to achieve the outcomes, but those with direct pharmacist-patient involvement resulted in the greatest A1C reductions (>1 percent decrease). Overall, most studies found that involving pharmacists in patient education was associated with at least a 0.5 percent reduction in A1C, a 17-18 mmHg reduction in blood pressure, and an 11 mg/dl reduction in LDL. The review authors caution that the findings are limited by flaws in study designs, including likely selection bias in the study populations. Only a few of the studies examined health care resource use. One reported that the average cost to lower A1C by 0.5 percent when utilizing a pharmacist was about $315 per patient, over approximately seven pharmacist visits.[95]

In a free-standing clinic, a pharmacist-provided program provides comprehensive diabetes and medication therapy management to the University of Kentucky's health plan members who have diabetes, primarily type 2. A study of 263 patients after one year of program participation found significant A1C and lipid improvements, increased screenings for diabetes complications, and increased patient satisfaction with care, compared with baseline. [96] A fee-for-service system is used.[97]

The Asheville Project—an employer collaboration

The Asheville Project was first implemented in 1997 as a pilot community-pharmacy care program, with 46 diabetes patients covered by two self-insured employers' health plans. Patients received education by CDEs and long-term community pharmacist follow-up using scheduled consultations, clinical assessment, goal setting, monitoring, and collaborative drug therapy management with physicians. Results showed a 50 percent reduction in sick days within 14 months that remained consistent after 5 years, and zero workers' compensation claims between 1997 and 2003. Mean A1C levels improved, and total mean direct medical costs decreased by $1,200 to $1,872 per patient per year compared with baseline.[98]

Case Study 7: Introducing Diabetes Education Services in Rural Communities

Gretchen Piatt, Ph.D.

Setting

The key goal of the Healthy People 2010 diabetes focus area is to increase the proportion of people with diabetes who receive formal diabetes education.[1] A common challenge in meeting this goal is generating referrals for diabetes outpatient education services.[2] To address this problem, the University of Pittsburgh Diabetes Institute (UPDI) implemented the Chronic Care Model[3] in a number of primary care practices in rural communities just outside of Pittsburgh, Pennsylvania.[4] The goal was to defragment the health system and restructure it to be evidence-based, population-based, and patient-centered.

Team members

Primary care physicians, office staff, and three CDEs (2 nurse CDEs and 1 dietitian CDE) are available on designated "diabetes days" in each of 17 primary care practices. The CDEs rotate to different offices based on their schedules.

Services

To increase referrals for education services, the UPDI began in 2003 to deliver diabetes self-management

education (DSME) at the point of service in the primary care office setting. The program started with four primary care practices and expanded to 17 throughout southwestern Pennsylvania. Decision-support tools, including the American Diabetes Association's (ADA's) Standards of Medical Care in Diabetes[5] and the National Standards for Diabetes Self-Management Education[6] were used by team members to provide consistent care and benchmarking to allow for clinical evaluation efforts. All DSME sessions used an empowerment approach to diabetes education, and clinical and behavioral outcomes were collected for each patient.

Communication

The CDEs met with the local practice physicians and their office staff to determine the best methods for communication and documentation within the practice and to arrange their appointment schedule.

Insurance coverage

Previous efforts have established that payment for DSME is critical in generating revenue to support the services of CDEs. In this setting, the CDEs secured ADA recognition for each of the 17 primary care sites and were then able to bill for their services in the primary care setting.

Continued on next page.

Today, more than 1,000 patients from five employers are enrolled for diabetes, asthma, and hypertension and lipid therapy management through the Asheville Project.

The Diabetes Ten City Challenge—an employer collaboration

Based on the Asheville Project model, the American Pharmacists Association (APhA) Foundation offers a non-profit consulting service under its Patient Self-Management Program for Diabetes, to help employers organize and implement diabetes management programs. The Diabetes Ten City Challenge is the latest initiative of the program in which participating employers offered a health care plan that waived co-payments for diabetes medications and supplies if patients worked with a pharmacist "coach" to monitor and manage their condition. In ten cities, thirty employers, hundreds of local pharmacists, and more than 800 people with diabetes participated in the initiative.

Results were reported for 573 patients with diabetes who had baseline and year-one medical and pharmacy claims and two or more documented visits with pharmacists. Statistically significant improvements were observed for key clinical measures, including A1C, LDL cholesterol, and mean systolic blood pressure. The rate of flu vaccinations and foot and eye exams increased. Employers realized an average annual savings of almost $1,100 in total health care costs per patient when compared to projected costs if the study had not been implemented, and participants saved an average of almost $600 per year.[99]

Podiatrists

Recent examples of successful multidisciplinary lower-extremity screening, prevention, and treatment programs for diabetes foot disease have been reported for managed care and a large military medical center.[73, 100] These programs significantly reduced amputation rates and foot-related hospital admissions. Teams involved podiatrists, vascular specialists, and other health care professionals.

Podiatrists and vascular surgeons play key roles in interdisciplinary lower-limb preservation teams that have significantly improved patient outcomes and reduced amputation rates in people with diabetes.[101, 102] Other team members may include trained physicians, primary care providers, nurses, footwear specialists, and others as necessary. Essential skills for these teams include assessment of the patient's vascular, neurological, and wound status; collection of soft tissue cultures and bone

---

Case Study 7: Introducing Diabetes Education Services in Rural Communities

Continued from page 28

Outcomes

Individuals who received DSME, both at the point of service and in traditional outpatient education settings experienced significant decreases in mean A1C levels over time (point of service DSME: 7.6 percent to 7.3 percent, p<0.0001; traditional DSME: 7.0 percent to 6.7 percent, p<0.0001); however, it must be noted that those who were referred to point-of-service DSME had higher baseline A1C values and may have represented people who needed more-specialized attention. The same pattern was observed in LDL-cholesterol levels. Individuals who received DSME at the point of service had significant declines in LDL (118 mg/dl to 101 mg/dl, p<0.0001). This decline was larger than was observed in individuals who received traditional outpatient DSME (116 mg/dl to 107 mg/dl, p<0.0001).

Related references

1. U.S. Department of Health and Human Services: Healthy People 2010. Washington D.C. U.S. Government Printing Office, 2000.

2. Balamurugan A, Rivera M., Jack L, Allen K, Morris S: Barriers to diabetes self-management education programs in underserved rural Arkansas: implications for program evaluation. Preventing Chronic Disease 2006; 3:1–8.

3. Wagner EH, Austin BT, Von Korff M: Organizing care for patients with chronic illness. Millbank Quarterly 1996; 74:511–544.

4. Siminerio, LM, Piatt GA, Emerson S, et al.: Deploying the chronic care model to implement and sustain diabetes self-management training programs. The Diabetes Educator 2006; 32(2): 253-60.

5. American Diabetes Association: Standards of medical care in diabetes–2011. Diabetes Care 2011; 34(Suppl 1): S11–61.

6. Funnell MM, Brown TL, Childs BP, et al.: National standards for diabetes self-management education. Diabetes Care 2007; 30(6): 1630–7.

biopsy; wound incision and debridement; initiation and modification of antibiotic therapy; and active monitoring of the healing phase. A hospital-based setting where such centers can provide both outpatient and inpatient care helps maintain a financially viable program.[103] A comprehensive microvascular complications checklist is being developed by the NDEP. (See NDEP Resources and **Case Study 8**.)

Case Study 8: A Podiatric Limb Preservation Team in Action

Vickie R. Driver, D.P.M.

Setting

The Limb Preservation Service at Madigan Army Medical Center in Tacoma, Washington, began as a "foot-at-risk" clinic in the Department of Podiatry. Over time, the foot-at-risk clinic specialized in the management of diabetes-related foot disease and became the Limb Preservation Service that provides both inpatient and outpatient services. The medical center is a 172-bed military regional tertiary care hospital with a beneficiary population of about 350,000. Madigan is one of three designated Level 2 trauma centers in the U.S. Medical Command.

Team members

The Limb Preservation Service is headed by the podiatry department. Clinic podiatrists conduct the first evaluation of patients with diabetes, assess risk factors, and manage foot ulcers and emergency treatment of foot infections. Vascular surgeons participate in the management of critical limb ischemia and peripheral arterial disease. A specialized wound care nurse assists the physician in carrying out wound care treatment plans. She or he also works independently as a wound care provider. A pedorthist provides customized shoe and orthotic devices.

Services

Regular care of the foot in patients with diabetes depends on the severity of their condition and the presence of risk factors. Patients followed by the limb preservation team receive comprehensive inpatient and outpatient care that includes
- state-of-the-art advanced wound care management
- medical and surgical management of infection
- at least a quarterly clinic visit (the frequency of the visits depends on the severity of the problem)
- ongoing education that includes families
- orthotic devices, extra-depth shoes, and custommade shoes as needed

A one-year randomized controlled trial compared usual medical care to usual care-plus-lifestyle case management provided by a registered dietitian. The case-managed group showed substantially greater weight loss, reduced A1C values, decreased prescription use, and increased health-related quality of life.[104] Case management participants had fewer inpatient admissions, which substantially lowered medical care costs.

Patient education is a high priority and is usually provided by a podiatrist or wound care nurse during both inpatient and outpatient visits. An individualized education plan is part of the electronic medical record. The higher the risk for limb loss, the more intensive the educational program.

Communication

Electronic medical records are used. Team members consult in person to discuss the most complex cases. Since it is an army medical center, specialist referrals are easily made and recommendations incorporated into the medical record. Two important factors contribute to the success of the limb preservation service: close collaboration among team members, and the fact that the patients remain within the military hospital system for a long period of time.

Insurance coverage

Patients pay for their care through TRICARE, the single-payer health care program of the United States Department of Defense Military Health System.

Outcomes

From the beginning of the Limb Preservation Service in 1999 to 2003, the rate of non-traumatic lower extremity amputations decreased significantly despite the increase in the overall population of patients with diabetes who were referred to the service.

Data were then collected on a random sample of 485 patients among the 8,422 patients with diabetes followed at the medical center between June 1999 and June 2004. Patients were stratified according to the University of Texas classification system that classifies diabetic wounds based on risk and severity and divided in two groups: those followed by the Limb Preservation Service and those followed by a non-specialized service. Over the five-year period, patients referred to the Limb Preservation Service had more severe disease than patients who were receiving non-specialized services. This resulted in a higher proportion of minor amputations in the Limb Preservation Service group but no significant increase in major amputations. *Continued on next page.*

Providing medical nutrition therapy to high-risk patients with type 2 diabetes and obesity decreased health plan costs by 34 percent.[105]

Registered nurses

With medical direction and defined protocols, nurses can make clinical management decisions about the treatment of diabetes, lipids, and hypertension; provide self-management education; and coordinate team services to meet the patient's health care needs. Compared to usual physician care, nurse-directed diabetes care for minority adults improved process measures 98 percent of the time compared to 54 percent; A1C levels decreased to 7 percent compared to 8.7 percent and 82 percent of patients met the LDL goal of <100mg/dl compared to 51 percent.[33]

One study evaluated the introduction of nurse case managers to collaborate at the office level with community-based primary care physicians in the care of 197 adult patients with type 2 diabetes. After six months, patients who received individual counseling, problem identification, care planning, and management recommendations from the nurse case manager had significantly improved mean systolic blood pressure and A1C values.[106]

A self-management program with a nurse case manager for children with diabetes showed improved A1C values, quality of life, and self-efficacy.[71] The frequency of nurse case manager follow-up contacts appears to be positively linked to better patient A1C values.[107]

Case Study 8: A Podiatric Limb Preservation Team in Action

Continued from page 30

Related references
Driver VR, Goodman RA, Fabbi M, et al.: The impact of a podiatric lead limb preservation team on disease outcomes and risk prediction in the diabetic lower extremity: a retrospective cohort study. J Am Podiatr Med Assoc 2010; 100(4): 235-41.

Driver VR: Reducing amputation rates in patients with diabetes in a military medical center. Diabetes Care 2005; 28(2): 248-53.

---

7. Summary

There is evidence that a team approach can reduce risk factors for type 2 diabetes, improve diabetes management, and lower the risk for chronic complications. This evidence supports an opportunity for health care professionals and organization leaders to help improve the health of people with diabetes. At the same time, it is important that studies of team interventions involving the skills of numerous health care professionals continue to elucidate effective ways to implement team care that improve patients' well-being and to assess the costs involved.

The commitment of an organization's leadership is essential for a team to provide comprehensive, lifetime management for patients with diabetes. Team care requires a collaborative, interactive, multi-skilled approach that maximizes the use of many different health professionals as educators, care coordinators, and providers of services to help patients achieve the best health outcomes possible. Community health workers, innovative interactions via telehealth technology, and alternative ways to deliver care such as group visits all contribute to the practice of team care. When patients participate as decision-making partners in care, improved diabetes control can be achieved. This improvement, in turn can, lead to greater patient satisfaction with care, better quality of life, improved health outcomes, and lower health care costs. Team care is likely to play a major role in future health care systems designed to provide comprehensive lifetime prevention and management of chronic diseases such as diabetes.

Appendix 1: Stratifying Care According to Patient Population Needs

Once the diabetes patient population is known, the team may want to stratify the population into groups according to the intensity of services required. Patients at risk for complications may require the lowest intensity of care and resources, whereas those with complications or comorbidities or those who are at break points in their disease management may require more-intensive services.

A. Identify patients at risk for type 2 diabetes

Risk factors for type 2 diabetes[40] include

- **Overweight adult:** Body Mass Index ≥25 kg/m2 (≥23 if Asian American or ≥26 if Pacific Islander) with one or more of the following
- **Family history:** has a first-degree relative with diabetes
- **Race/Ethnicity:** African American, Hispanic/Latino, American Indian and Alaska Native, or Asian American and Pacific Islander
- **History of gestational diabetes** or gave birth to a baby weighing > 9 lbs
- **Hypertension:** blood pressure >140/90
- **Abnormal lipid levels:** HDL cholesterol level <35mg/dl; triglyceride level >250 mg/dl
- **IGT or IFG:** on previous testing
- **Signs of insulin resistance:** such as acanthosis nigricans or polycystic ovarian syndrome (PCOS)
- **History of vascular disease:** diagnosed by physical exam and testing
- **Inactive lifestyle:** is physically active less than three times a week

In the absence of the above risk factors, people age 45 and older are considered at risk and should be tested at least at three-year intervals.

B. Identify patients at risk for diabetes complications

Identifying patients at risk for diabetes complications can help the team to effectively stratify services. Clinical information to assess risk includes

- A1C values
- blood pressure control
- lipid control
- cardiovascular disease risk
- eye disease risk
- foot disease risk
- evidence of increased urinary albumin excretion and/or reduced eGFR
- smoking habits
- alcohol use
- family history of diabetes complications including premature cardiovascular disease
- duration of the disease
- oral exam status
- hypoglycemia history
- depression and other psychosocial illness
- reduced literacy
- inadequate social support

Patients with type 2 diabetes who are largely free of diabetes complications or other comorbidities will benefit from relatively low-cost preventive care focused on risk factor reduction and health promotion. After screening for complications, the team could offer group discussions about risk factor reduction and self-management issues such as nutrition, weight management, and ways to incorporate regular physical activity into lifestyles.

C. Identify patients with complications and other comorbidities

Identifying the patients who have diabetes complications or other comorbidities can help determine those who will require more extensive resources, such as allocation of additional team members, more aggressive protocol management, or more frequent follow-up.[108, 109] Analyses of administrative databases have demonstrated that a large fraction of health care dollars are allocated to a small proportion of the population with multiple comorbidities. It is important to note, however, that patients with complications are an evolving group and that for practical planning purposes, periodic reassessment is essential.

D. Identify patients at "break points"

To predict other potential high resource users, identifying patients at "break points" in the course of their disease may be helpful. These points include

- new onset of type 1 or type 2 diabetes
- A1C consistently above 8 percent
- new onset of significant complications
- frequent or severe hypoglycemia
- pregnancy in a woman with diabetes
- initiation of insulin therapy[27]

Assessing reasons for consistently elevated A1C values in the patient population also may help team planning. The level of diabetes control can be affected by several factors

- limited provider availability and service payment
- outdated or ineffective management protocols
- limited medical and dental insurance coverage for patients
- limited insurance coverage for medications or supplies
- cognitive, psychological, and social barriers that limit patient participation in diabetes management
- limited diabetes self-management education or self-management support

Appendix 2: Scope of Practice for Diabetes Educators and Board-Certified Advanced Diabetes Management Practitioners

A. Guidelines and Competencies

Guidelines for the Practice of Diabetes Education delineates the roles and responsibilities for individuals and organizations involved in the facilitation and delivery of diabetes education and care for persons with or at risk for diabetes and their families/caregivers.

www.diabeteseducator.org/DiabetesEducation/position/Practice_Guidelines.html

Competencies for Diabetes Educators provides a master list of the knowledge and skills needed for the various levels of practice. They are the basis for education, training, development, and performance appraisal of all clinicians engaged in diabetes education.

www.diabeteseducator.org/export/sites/aade/_resources/pdf/competencies.pdf

B. The Role of Diabetes Educators

Diabetes educators help people with and at risk for diabetes and related conditions to achieve behavior-change goals that lead to better clinical outcomes and improved health status. Diabetes educators apply in-depth knowledge and skills in the biological and social sciences, communication, counseling, and education to provide self-management education and training.

www.diabeteseducator.org/export/sites/aade/_resources/pdf/Definition_Diabetes_Educator.pdf

Certified Diabetes Educators (CDE) receive certification from the National Certification Board for Diabetes Educators by taking a voluntary examination that indicates distinct and specialized knowledge in diabetes patient self-management education, thereby promoting high-quality care for people with diabetes. Objectives of the certification program are to

- provide a mechanism to demonstrate professional accomplishment and growth

- provide formal recognition of specialty practice and knowledge at a mastery level
- provide validation of dedication to diabetes education to consumers and employers
- promote continuing commitment to best practices, current standards, and knowledge

www.ncbde.org

Certification can be awarded to those who meet eligibility requirements and are from the following disciplines: registered dietitian, exercise physiologist, health educator, registered nurse, nutritionist, occupational therapist, optometrist, pharmacist, physical therapist, physician (M.D. or D.O.), physician assistant, podiatrist, public health professional, clinical psychologist, or social worker.

www.ncbde.org/certification_info/eligibility-requirements

C. The Role of Board-Certified Advanced Diabetes Management (BC-ADM) Practitioners

The Board-Certified Advanced Diabetes Manager (BC-ADM) credential was developed to verify clinical care skills among advanced practitioners. The BC-ADM credential is a multidisciplinary credential for nurses, dietitians, and pharmacists who have advanced degrees. It is different from the CDE credential in that it focuses on advanced clinical management of diabetes. The exam covers the domains of clinical practice, collaboration, research, patient and professional diabetes education, and public and community health.

www.diabeteseducator.org/ProfessionalResources/Certification/BC-ADM

Appendix 3: Quality Improvement Indicators for Diabetes Care

The increasing demand for high-quality care from managed health care systems, payers, and the public is an important development. The Diabetes Quality Improvement Project was an initial national collaborative effort to improve diabetes care and the quality of life for people with diabetes, consisting of eight performance measures for diabetes care that cover A1C and lipid testing and assessment of the eyes, kidneys, and feet. Numerous public agencies (the Department of Defense, the Health Care Financing Administration, multiple state Medicaid programs, the Indian Health Service, and the Veterans Health Administration) and private groups (the National Committee for Quality Assurance, NCQA) have developed quality measures in comprehensive diabetes care.

Diabetes performance measures have been incorporated into NCQA's HEDIS* measures; these are reported publicly for Medicare, Medicaid, and commercial and managed care plans that serve Medicare beneficiaries. The Diabetes Recognition Program (DRP) administered by NCQA, is a voluntary recognition program for physicians and nurse practitioners who demonstrate high-quality outpatient diabetes care. A number of the processes and outcomes measured in the DRP could readily involve team care (see *www.ncqa.org*).

*Healthcare Effectiveness Data and Information Set

Diabetes HEDIS measures for care, screening, or testing needed for comprehensive diabetes care for adults ages 18 to 75, consist of the following

- A1C testing twice a year
- A1C result > 9% = poor control measure
- A1C < 8%
- A1C result < 7% = good control measure
- LDL-C measurement
- LDL-C result < 100
- retinal eye exam
- nephropathy screening test or evidence of nephropathy
- blood pressure < 140/90
- blood pressure < 130/80

Appendix 4: Medicare for People with Diabetes

What Is Medicare?

Medicare is health insurance for people age 65 or older, under age 65 with certain disabilities, and any age with end-stage renal disease (permanent kidney failure requiring dialysis or a kidney transplant). People with diabetes who are eligible for Medicare can get the most from their Medicare benefits by learning about the types of services that are available. People with diabetes are encouraged to ask their health care team about the benefits they qualify for and visit www.medicare.gov to get specific details from Medicare.

What Benefits Does Medicare Offer for People with Diabetes?

People with diabetes enrolled in Medicare may be covered for all or part of the cost for
- a "Welcome to Medicare" physical exam when they enroll
- A1C testing
- cholesterol testing
- diabetes self-management training to learn how to manage diabetes
- medical nutrition therapy: nutrition and lifestyle assessments, diet management information, and nutrition counseling
- diabetes equipment and supplies for self-monitoring of blood glucose, including special equipment for persons with low vision
- foot exams by a podiatrist if medically necessary
- therapeutic shoes and inserts if medically necessary
- a dilated eye exam and glaucoma screening
- flu and pneumonia shots
- diabetes medications
- insulin pumps
- kidney function tests

What Benefits Does Medicare Offer for People At Risk for Diabetes?

People enrolled in Medicare who are at risk for type 2 diabetes may be covered for all or part of the cost of
- a "Welcome to Medicare" physical exam when they enroll
- yearly diabetes screening for people who are at risk for diabetes and twice yearly screening for people diagnosed with prediabetes (people are considered at risk if they have any of the following: high blood pressure, history of abnormal cholesterol and triglyceride levels, obesity, or a history of high blood glucose)
- cholesterol screening—every five years

To learn more

1-800-MEDICARE (1-800-633-4227), in English and Spanish
TTY/TDD 1-877-486-2048

Medicare and You
http://www.medicare.gov/Publications/Pubs/pdf/10050.pdf

Medicare Coverage of Diabetes Supplies and Services
http://www.medicare.gov/Publications/Pubs/pdf/11022.pdf

Medicare Information for Caregivers
http://www.medicare.gov/caregivers/

Team Care-Related Resources

National Diabetes Education Program
www.YourDiabetesInfo.org

- Diabetes HealthSense
- Diabetes Numbers At-a-Glance card
- Diabetes at Work
- Feet Can Last a Lifetime: A Health Care Provider's Guide to Preventing Foot Problems
- Guiding Principles for Diabetes Care
- Systems Change for Better Diabetes Care Models, links, and tools to help health care professionals implement systems change
- Transitions—From Pediatric to Adult Health Care
- Working Together to Manage Diabetes: A Guide for Pharmacists, Podiatrists, Optometrists, and Dental Professionals, 2007

American Academy of Family Physicians
www.aafp.org

- Patient-Centered Medical Home
- CD-9 Coding Tools from Family Practice Medicine

American Academy of Pediatrics
www.aap.org

- Patient-Centered Medical Home

American Association of Clinical Endocrinologists
www.aace.com

- AACE Online Endocrine Coding Manual

American Association of Diabetes Educators
www.diabeteseducator.org

- AADE 7
- Online learning modules about Medicare DSMT and MNT payment provided in a variety of practice settings
- Ask the Reimbursement Expert (a free benefit for AADE members–login required)
- Education program accreditation
- Reimbursement Tips for Primary Care Practice, revised 2009
- Position Statement: Community Health Workers in Diabetes Management and Prevention
- Guidelines for the Practice of Diabetes Education
- Competencies for Diabetes Educators

American College of Physicians
www.acponline.org

- ACP Diabetes Care Guide: A Team-Based Practice Manual and Self-assessment Program
- Patient-Centered Medical Home

American Diabetes Association
www.diabetes.org

- Standards of Medical Care in Diabetes – 2010 (updated yearly)
- National Standards for Diabetes Self-Management Education[31]
- The ADA Education Recognition Program Application

Academy of Nutrition and Dietetics

www.eatright.org

- Diabetes MNT reimbursement resources and information
- The Diabetes Care and Education (DCE) Practice Group professional resources
- DCE free, reproducible patient education materials

American Optometric Association

www.aoa.org

- American Optometric Association: Role of Retinal Imaging and Comprehensive Eye Examinations in the Care of Patients with Diabetes, June 2008
- Diabetic Eye Examination Report Form

American Pharmacists Association

www.pharmacist.com

- American Pharmacists Association Foundation
- Asheville Project
- Diabetes Ten City Challenge

American Telemedicine Association

www.americantelemed.org

- The American Telemedicine Association Telehealth Practice Recommendations for Diabetic Retinopathy: A Roadmap of Technical Standards, Clinical Guidelines, and Administrative Procedures, 2004

Centers for Disease Control and Prevention

http://www.cdc.org

- Community Health Workers/Promotores de Salud: Critical Connections in Communities

Centers for Medicare and Medicaid Services (CMS)

www.cms.gov

- Requirements for reimbursement of diabetes self-management training
- CMS rules for MNT reimbursement
- Medicare coverage for people for people with or at risk for diabetes
- Quick Reference Information: Medicare Preventive Services

Indian Health Service

www.ihs.gov

- The Indian Health Service (IHS)-Joslin Vision Network Teleophthalmology Program

International Diabetes Federation

www.idf.org

- Diabetes Education Modules

Peer Support

www.peersforprogress.org

- World Health Organization (2007). Peer Support Programs in Diabetes
- Peers for Progress
- California Healthcare Foundation, Building Peer Support Programs: Seven Models for Success

Veterans Affairs

www.va.gov

- Diabetes Program
- National Veterans Rural Health Resource Center
- VHA Directive 2006-050: Preservation—Amputation Care and Treatment (PACT)

References

1. Centers for Disease Control and Prevention: National diabetes fact sheet: general information and national estimates on diabetes in the United States, 2011. Atlanta, GA: U.S. Department of Health and Human Services, Centers for Disease Control and Prevention, 2011.

2. Fagot-Campagna A, Pettitt DJ, Engelgau MM, et al.: Type 2 diabetes among North American children and adolescents: an epidemiologic review and a public health perspective. J Pediatr 2000; 136(5): 664-72.

3. Nathan DM, Cleary PA, Backlund JY, et al.: Intensive diabetes treatment and cardiovascular disease in patients with type 1 diabetes. N Engl J Med 2005; 353(25): 2643-53.

4. Holman RR, Paul SK, Bethel MA, et al.: 10-year follow-up of intensive glucose control in type 2 diabetes. N Engl J Med 2008; 359(15): 1577-89.

5. American Diabetes Association: Economic costs of diabetes in the U.S. in 2007. Diabetes Care 2008; 31(3): 596-615.

6. Herman WH, Eastman RC: The effects of treatment on the direct costs of diabetes. Diabetes Care 1998; 21 Suppl 3: C19-24.

7. Gilmer TP, O'Connor PJ, Manning WG, et al.: The cost to health plans of poor glycemic control. Diabetes Care 1997; 20(12): 1847-53.

8. Knowler WC, Barrett-Connor E, Fowler SE, et al.: Reduction in the incidence of type 2 diabetes with lifestyle intervention or metformin. N Engl J Med 2002; 346(6): 393-403.

9. Herman WH, Hoerger TJ, Brandle M, et al.: The cost-effectiveness of lifestyle modification or metformin in preventing type 2 diabetes in adults with impaired glucose tolerance. Ann Intern Med 2005; 142(5): 323-32.

10. Knowler WC, Fowler SE, Hamman RF, et al.: 10-year follow-up of diabetes incidence and weight loss in the Diabetes Prevention Program Outcomes Study. Lancet 2009; 374(9702): 1677-86.

11. Wagner EH: Chronic disease management: What will it take to improve care for chronic illness? Effective Clinical Practice 1998; 1: 2-4.

12. Bodenheimer T, Wagner EH, Grumbach K: Improving primary care for patients with chronic illness. JAMA 2002; 288(14): 1775-9.

13. Carrier E, Gourevitch MN, Shah NR: Medical homes: challenges in translating theory into practice. Med Care 2009; 47(7): 714-22.

14. Erickson CD, Splett PL, Mullett SS, et al.: The healthy learner model for student chronic condition management—part I. J Sch Nurs 2006; 22(6): 310-8.

15. Peterson KA, Radosevich DM, O'Connor PJ, et al.: Improving Diabetes Care in Practice: findings from the TRANSLATE trial. Diabetes Care 2008; 31(12): 2238-43.

16. American Academy of Physician Assistants: 2008 AAPA Physician Assistant Census Report. Alexandria, VA, 2009.

17. Cooper RA: New directions for nurse practitioners and physician assistants in the era of physician shortages. Acad Med 2007; 82(9): 827-8.

18. Goolsby MJ: 2004 AANP National Nurse Practitioner Sample Survey, part I: an overview. J Am Acad Nurse Pract 2005; 17(9): 337-41.

19. Roman SH, Harris MI: Management of diabetes mellitus from a public health perspective. Endocrinol Metab Clin North Am 1997; 26(3): 443-74.

20. Bodenheimer T, Wagner EH, Grumbach K: Improving primary care for patients with chronic illness: the chronic care model, Part 2. JAMA 2002; 288(15): 1909-14.

21. Tsai AC, Morton SC, Mangione CM, et al.: A meta-analysis of interventions to improve care for chronic illnesses. Am J Manag Care 2005; 11(8): 478-88.

22. Robert Graham Center: The Patient Centered Medical Home History, Seven Core Features, Evidence and Transformational Change. Washington, DC: Policy Studies in Family Medicine and Primary Care, 2007.

23. Reid RJ, Coleman K, Johnson EA, et al.: The group health medical home at year two: cost savings, higher patient satisfaction, and less burnout for providers. Health Aff (Millwood); 29(5): 835-43.

24. Multi-payer Advanced Primary Care Practice (MAPCP) Demonstration Fact Sheet. *www.cms. gov/DemoProjectsEvalRpts/downloads/mapcdemo_ Factsheet.pdf*

25. O'Connor PJ, Sperl-Hillen JM: The role of diabetes educators in the medical home. Diabetes Spectrum 2009; 22(2): 124-6.

26. Erickson CD, Splett PL, Mullett SS, et al.: The healthy learner model for student chronic condition management—part II: the asthma initiative. J Sch Nurs 2006; 22(6): 319-29.

27. Quickel KE, Jr.: Managed care and diabetes, with special attention to the issue of who should provide care. Trans Am Clin Climatol Assoc 1996; 108: 184-95.

28. Scanlon DP, Hollenbeak CS, Beich J, et al.: Financial and clinical impact of team-based treatment for Medicaid enrollees with diabetes in a federally qualified health center. Diabetes Care 2008; 31(11): 2160-5.

29. Huang ES, Zhang Q, Brown SE, et al.: The cost-effectiveness of improving diabetes care in U.S. federally qualified community health centers. Health Serv Res 2007; 42(6 Pt 1): 2174-93; discussion 2294-323.

30. Ray MD: Shared borders: achieving the goals of interdisciplinary patient care. Am J Health Syst Pharm 1998; 55(13): 1369-74.

31. Funnell MM, Brown TL, Childs BP, et al.: National standards for diabetes self-management education. Diabetes Care 2007; 30(6): 1630-7.

32. Shojania KG, Ranji SR, McDonald KM, et al.: Effects of quality improvement strategies for type 2 diabetes on glycemic control: a meta-regression analysis. JAMA 2006; 296(4): 427-40.

33. Davidson MB, Castellanos M, Duran P, et al.: Effective diabetes care by a registered nurse following treatment algorithms in a minority population. Am J Manag Care 2006; 12(4): 226-32.

34. Silverstein JH, Rosenbloom AL: Treatment of type 2 diabetes mellitus in children and adolescents. J Pediatr Endocrinol Metab 2000; 13(Suppl 6): 1403-9.

35. Brink SJ, Miller M, Moltz KC: Education and multidisciplinary team care concepts for pediatric and adolescent diabetes mellitus. J Pediatr Endocrinol Metab 2002; 15(8): 1113-30.

36. Gaede P, Vedel P, Larsen N, et al.: Multifactorial intervention and cardiovascular disease in patients with type 2 diabetes. N Engl J Med 2003; 348(5): 383-93.

37. Gaede P, Lund-Andersen H, Parving HH, et al.: Effect of a multifactorial intervention on mortality in type 2 diabetes. N Engl J Med 2008; 358(6): 580-91.

38. Hastings C: The changing multidisciplinary team. Nurs Econ 1997; 15(2): 106-8, 105.

39. Engelgau MM, Geiss LS, Manninen DL, et al.: Use of services by diabetes patients in managed care organizations. Development of a diabetes surveillance system. CDC Diabetes in Managed Care Work Group. Diabetes Care 1998; 21(12): 2062-8.

40. American Diabetes Association: Standards of medical care in diabetes—2011. Diabetes Care 2011; 34(Suppl 1): S11-61.

41. Sarkar U, Handley MA, Gupta R, et al.: Use of an interactive, telephone-based self-management support program to identify adverse events among ambulatory diabetes patients. J Gen Intern Med 2008; 23(4): 459-65.

42. Fursse J, Clarke M, Jones R, et al.: Early experience in using telemonitoring for the management of chronic disease in primary care. J Telemed Telecare 2008; 14(3): 122-4.

43. Piette JD, McPhee SJ, Weinberger M, et al.: Use of automated telephone disease management calls in an ethnically diverse sample of low-income patients with diabetes. Diabetes Care 1999; 22(8): 1302-9.

44. Adkins JW, Storch EA, Lewin AB, et al.: Home-based behavioral health intervention: Use of a telehealth model to address poor adherence to type-1 diabetes medical regimens. Telemed J E Health 2006; 12(3): 370-2.

45. Ferris FL, 3rd: Photocoagulation for diabetic retinopathy. Early Treatment Diabetic Retinopathy Study Research Group. JAMA 1991; 266(9): 1263-5.

46. Robinson C: Telemedicine: An emerging technology. One the Cutting Edge; Diabetes Care & Education; American Dietetic Association 2007; 27(6).

47. Scott JC, Conner DA, Venohr I, et al.: Effectiveness of a group outpatient visit model for chronically ill older health maintenance organization members: a 2-year randomized trial of the cooperative health care clinic. J Am Geriatr Soc 2004; 52(9): 1463-70.

48. Kirsh S, Watts S, Pascuzzi K, et al.: Shared medical appointments based on the chronic care model: a quality improvement project to address the challenges of patients with diabetes with high cardiovascular risk. Qual Saf Health Care 2007; 16(5): 349-53.

49. Wagner EH, Grothaus LC, Sandhu N, et al.: Chronic care clinics for diabetes in primary care: a system-wide randomized trial. Diabetes Care 2001; 24(4): 695-700.

50. Trento M, Passera P, Borgo E, et al.: A 5-year randomized controlled study of learning, problem solving ability, and quality of life modifications in people with type 2 diabetes managed by group care. Diabetes Care 2004; 27(3): 670-5.

51. Clancy DE, Cope DW, Magruder KM, et al.: Evaluating group visits in an uninsured or inadequately insured patient population with uncontrolled type 2 diabetes. Diabetes Educ 2003; 29(2): 292-302.

52. Deakin T, McShane CE, Cade JE, et al.: Group based training for self-management strategies in people with type 2 diabetes mellitus. Cochrane Database Syst Rev 2005(2): CD003417.

53. Davies MJ, Heller S, Skinner TC, et al.: Effectiveness of the diabetes education and self management for ongoing and newly diagnosed (DESMOND) programme for people with newly diagnosed type 2 diabetes: cluster randomised controlled trial. BMJ 2008; 336(7642): 491-5.

54. Gage H, Hampson S, Skinner TC, et al.: Educational and psychosocial programmes for adolescents with diabetes: approaches, outcomes and cost-effectiveness. Patient Educ Couns 2004; 53(3): 333-46.

55. Hampson SE, Skinner TC, Hart J, et al.: Effects of educational and psychosocial interventions for adolescents with diabetes mellitus: a systematic review. Health Technol Assess 2001; 5(10): 1-79.

56. Klonoff DC, Schwartz DM: An economic analysis of interventions for diabetes. Diabetes Care 2000; 23(3): 390-404.

57. Loveman E, Cave C, Green C, et al.: The clinical and cost-effectiveness of patient education models for diabetes: a systematic review and economic evaluation. Health Technol Assess 2003; 7(22): iii, 1-190.

58. Norris SL, Nichols PJ, Caspersen CJ, et al.: Increasing diabetes self-management education in community settings. A systematic review. Am J Prev Med 2002; 22(4 Suppl): 39-66.

59. Boren SA, Fitzner KA, Panhalkar PS, et al.: Costs and benefits associated with diabetes education: a review of the literature. Diabetes Educ 2009; 35(1): 72-96.

60. Robbins JM, Thatcher GE, Webb DA, et al.: Nutritionist visits, diabetes classes, and hospitalization rates and charges: the Urban Diabetes Study. Diabetes Care 2008; 31(4): 655-60.

61. Duncan I, Birkmeyer C, Coughlin S, et al.: Assessing the value of diabetes education. Diabetes Educ 2009; 35(5): 752-60.

62. Kilpatrick KE, Brownson CA: Building the business case for diabetes self management: a handbook for program managers. St. Louis: Diabetes Initiative, National Program Office at Washington University School of Medicine, 2008.

63. Brownson CA, O'Toole ML, Gowri S, et al.: Clinic-community partnerships: A foundation for providing community supports for diabetes care and self-management. Diabetes Spectrum 2007; 20(4): 209-214.

64. Finch EA, Kelly MS, Marrero DG, et al.: Training YMCA wellness instructors to deliver an adapted version of the Diabetes Prevention Program lifestyle intervention. Diabetes Educ 2009; 35(2): 224-8, 232.

65. Ackermann RT, Finch EA, Brizendine E, et al.: Translating the Diabetes Prevention Program into the community. The DEPLOY Pilot Study. Am J Prev Med 2008; 35(4): 357-63.

66. Janicke DM, Sallinen BJ, Perri MG, et al.: Comparison of parent-only vs family-based interventions for overweight children in underserved rural settings: outcomes from project STORY. Arch Pediatr Adolesc Med 2008; 162(12): 1119-25.

67. Janicke DM, Sallinen BJ, Perri MG, et al.: Comparison of program costs for parent-only and family-based interventions for pediatric obesity in medically underserved rural settings. J Rural Health 2009; 25(3): 326-30.

68. Norris SL, Chowdhury FM, Van Le K, et al.: Effectiveness of community health workers in the care of persons with diabetes. Diabet Med 2006; 23(5): 544-56.

69. Heisler M: Building peer suport programs: Seven models for success. Oakland, CA: California Healthcare Foundation, 2006.

70. Domurat ES: Diabetes managed care and clinical outcomes: the Harbor City, California Kaiser Permanente diabetes care system. Am J Manag Care 1999; 5(10): 1299-307.

71. Caravalho JY, Saylor CR: An evaluation of a nurse case-managed program for children with diabetes. Pediatr Nurs 2000; 26(3): 296-300, 328.

72. Marshall CL, Bluestein M, Briere E, et al.: Improving outpatient diabetes management through a collaboration of six competing, capitated Medicare managed care plans. Am J Med Qual 2000; 15(2): 65-71.

73. Driver VR, Madsen J, Goodman RA: Reducing amputation rates in patients with diabetes at a military medical center: the limb preservation service model. Diabetes Care 2005; 28(2): 248-53.

74. Rith-Najarian S, Dannels E, Acton K: Preventing amputations from diabetes mellitus: the Indian Health Service experience. West Indian Med J 2001; 50 Suppl 1: 41-3.

75. Frykberg RG: Diabetic foot ulcerations: management and adjunctive therapy. Clin Podiatr Med Surg 2003; 20(4): 709-28.

76. Wrobel JS, Charns MP, Diehr P, et al.: The relationship between provider coordination and diabetes-related foot outcomes. Diabetes Care 2003; 26(11): 3042-7.

77. Haase R, Russell S: Improving diabetes care and outcomes in a rural primary care clinic. Jt Comm J Qual Patient Saf 2006; 32(5): 246-52.

78. Siminerio LM, Piatt G, Zgibor JC: Implementing the chronic care model for improvements in diabetes care and education in a rural primary care practice. Diabetes Educ 2005; 31(2): 225-34.

79. Litaker D, Mion L, Planavsky L, et al.: Physician - nurse practitioner teams in chronic disease management: the impact on costs, clinical effectiveness, and patients' perception of care. J Interprof Care 2003; 17(3): 223-37.

80. Solberg LI, Klevan DH, Asche SE: Crossing the quality chasm for diabetes care: the power of one physician, his team, and systems thinking. J Am Board Fam Med 2007; 20(3): 299-306.

81. Ginsberg BH, Tan MH, Mazze R, et al.: Staged diabetes management: computerizing a disease state management program. J Med Syst 1998; 22(2): 77-87.

82. Hirsch IB, Goldberg HI, Ellsworth A, et al.: A multifaceted intervention in support of diabetes treatment guidelines: a cont trial. Diabetes Res Clin Pract 2002; 58(1): 27-36.

83. International Diabetes Federation Clinical GuidelinesTask Force: IDF Guideline on oral health for people with diabetes. Brussels, 2009.

84. Albert DA, Sadowsky D, Papapanou P, et al.: An examination opopulation. BMC Health Serv Res 2006; 6: 103.

85. Eke PI, Genco RJ: CDC Periodontal Disease Surveillance Project: background, objectives, and progress report. J Periodontol 2007; 78(7 Suppl): 1366-71.

86. World Health Organization: Report on the Global Tobacco Epidemic: the MPOWER package. Geneva, 2008.

87. Katon W, Unutzer J, Fan MY, et al.: Cost-effectiveness and net benefit of enhanced treatment of depression for older adults with diabetes and depression. Diabetes Care 2006; 29(2): 265-70.

88. Hunkeler EM, Katon W, Tang L, et al.: Long term outcomes from the IMPACT randomised trial for depressed elderly patients in primary care. BMJ 2006; 332(7536): 259-63.

89. Mukhtar Q, Jack L, Jr., Martin M, et al.: Evaluating progress toward Healthy People 2010 national diabetes objectives. Prev Chronic Dis 2006; 3(1): A11.

90. Aiello LP, Cahill MT, Wong JS: Systemic considerations in the management of diabetic retinopathy. Am J Ophthalmol 2001; 132(5): 760-76.

91. Winters JE, Messner LV, Gable EM, et al.: Coordinating eye and primary medical care in a low-income and uninsured population: the experience of the Vision of Hope Health Alliance. Optometry 2008; 79(12): 730-6.

92. Persaud DD, Jreige S, LeBlanc RP: Enhancing vision care integration: 1. Development of practice algorithms. Can J Ophthalmol 2004; 39(3): 219-24.

93. Jones SL, Nichols KK: Diabetic eye examination report. Optometry 2007; 78(11): 588-95.

94. Siminerio LM, Piatt GA, Emerson S, et al.: Deploying the chronic care model to implement and sustain diabetes self-management training programs. Diabetes Educ 2006; 32(2): 253-60.

95. Wubben DP, Vivian EM: Effects of pharmacist outpatient interventions on adults with diabetes mellitus: a systematic review. Pharmacotherapy 2008; 28(4): 421-36.

96. Johnson CL, Nicholas A, Divine H, et al.: Outcomes from DiabetesCARE: a pharmacist-provided diabetes management service. J Am Pharm Assoc (2003) 2008; 48(6): 722-30.

97. Divine H, Nicholas A, Johnson CL, et al.: PharmacistCARE: description of a pharmacist care service and lessons learned along the way. J Am Pharm Assoc (2003) 2008; 48(6): 793-802.

98. Cranor CW, Bunting BA, Christensen DB: The Asheville Project: long-term clinical and economic outcomes of a community pharmacy diabetes care program. J Am Pharm Assoc (Wash) 2003; 43(2): 173-84.

99. Fera T, Bluml BM, Ellis WM: Diabetes Ten City Challenge: final economic and clinical results. J Am Pharm Assoc (2003) 2009; 49(3): 383-91.

100. Lavery LA, Wunderlich RP, Tredwell JL: Disease management for the diabetic foot: effectiveness of a diabetic foot prevention program to reduce amputations and hospitalizations. Diabetes Res Clin Pract 2005; 70(1): 31-7.

101. Fitzgerald RH, Mills JL, Joseph W, et al.: The diabetic rapid response acute foot team: 7 essential skills for targeted limb salvage. Eplasty 2009; 9: e15.

102. Sumpio BE, Armstrong DG, Lavery LA, et al.: The role of interdisciplinary team approach in the management of the diabetic foot: a joint statement from the Society for Vascular Surgery and the American Podiatric Medical Association. J Vasc Surg 2010; 51(6): 1504-6.

103. Attinger CE, Hoang H, Steinberg J, et al.: How to make a hospital-based wound center financially viable: the Georgetown University Hospital model. Gynecol Oncol 2008; 111(2 Suppl): S92-7.

104. Wolf AM, Conaway MR, Crowther JQ, et al.: Translating lifestyle intervention to practice in obese patients with type 2 diabetes: Improving Control with Activity and Nutrition (ICAN) study. Diabetes Care 2004; 27(7): 1570-6.

105. Wolf AM, Siadaty M, Yaeger B, et al.: Effects of lifestyle intervention on health care costs: Improving Control with Activity and Nutrition (ICAN). J Am Diet Assoc 2007; 107(8): 1365-73.

106. Hiss RG, Armbruster BA, Gillard ML, et al.: Nurse care manager collaboration with community-based physicians providing diabetes care: a randomized controlled trial. Diabetes Educ 2007; 33(3): 493-502.

107. Polonsky WH, Earles J, Smith S, et al.: Integrating medical management with diabetes self-management training: a randomized control trial of the Diabetes Outpatient Intensive Treatment program. Diabetes Care 2003; 26(11): 3048-53.

108. Newton KM, Wagner EH, Ramsey SD, et al.: The use of automated data to identify complications and comorbidities of diabetes: a validation study. J Clin Epidemiol 1999; 52(3): 199-207.

109. Selby JV, Karter AJ, Ackerson LM, et al.: Developing a prediction rule from automate clinical databases to identify high-risk patients in a large population with diabetes. Diabetes Care 2001; 24(9): 1547-55.

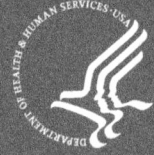 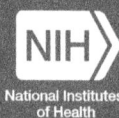 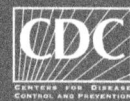

The U.S. Department of Health and Human Services' National Diabetes Education Program (NDEP) is jointly sponsored by the National Institutes of Health and the Centers for Disease Control and Prevention with the support of more than 200 partner organizations.

Participants in clinical trials can play a more active role in their own health care, gain access to new research treatments before they are widely available, and help others by contributing to medical research.

For information about current studies, visit www.ClinicalTrials.gov.

www.YourDiabetesInfo.org

1-888-693-NDEP (1-888-693-6337)

TTY: 1-866-569-1162

NIH Publication No. 13-7739

NDEP-37

Last Reviewed February 2013

NIDDK prints on recycled paper with bio-based ink.

www.ingramcontent.com/pod-product-compliance
Lightning Source LLC
Chambersburg PA
CBHW080342290526
45791CB00009BA/2706